Nutrient Timing

Fueling Strategies to Unlock Peak Performance

Lauren Link, MS, RD, CSSD

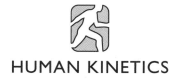

HUMAN KINETICS

Library of Congress Cataloging-in-Publication Data

Names: Link, Lauren, author.
Title: Nutrient timing : fueling strategies to unlock peak performance /
    Lauren Link.
Description: Champaign, IL : Human Kinetics, [2025] | Includes
    bibliographical references and index.
Identifiers: LCCN 2023038334 (print) | LCCN 2023038335 (ebook) | ISBN
    9781718218031 (paperback) | ISBN 9781718218048 (epub) | ISBN
    9781718218055 (pdf)
Subjects: LCSH: Athletes—Nutrition. | BISAC: HEALTH & FITNESS / Diet &
    Nutrition / Nutrition | SPORTS & RECREATION / Training
Classification: LCC TX361.A8 L485 2025 (print) | LCC TX361.A8 (ebook) |
    DDC 613.2—dc23/eng/20231116
LC record available at https://lccn.loc.gov/2023038334
LC ebook record available at https://lccn.loc.gov/2023038335

ISBN: 978-1-7182-1803-1 (print)

Copyright © 2025 by Lauren Link

Acquisitions Editor: Korey Van Wyk; **Developmental Editor:** Anne Hall; **Managing Editor:** Shawn Donnelly; **Copyeditor:** Heather Gauen Hutches; **Indexer:** Rebecca L. McCorkle; **Permissions Manager:** Laurel Mitchell; **Graphic Designer:** Julie L. Denzer; **Cover Designer:** Keri Evans; **Cover Design Specialist:** Susan Rothermel Allen; **Photograph (cover):** Simonkr/E+/Getty Images; **Photographs (interior):** © Human Kinetics, unless otherwise noted; **Photo Asset Manager:** Laura Fitch; **Photo Production Manager:** Jason Allen **Senior Art Manager:** Kelly Hendren; **Production:** MPS; **Printer:** Versa Press

Human Kinetics   *United States and International*   *Canada*
1607 N. Market Street   Website: **US.HumanKinetics.com**   Website: **Canada.HumanKinetics.com**
Champaign, IL 61820   Email: info@hkusa.com   Email: info@hkcanada.com
USA   Phone: 1-800-747-4457

E8936

As I was writing this book, I didn't especially think I would have a dedication. To be honest, there was no one in particular who inspired me or for whom I felt especially inspired to write it. However, in the final weeks of the editing process, my work family was dealt a devastating blow with the sudden and incredibly unexpected passing of my boss, my mentor, and my friend, Doug Boersma. As I sat in front of my computer trying desperately to focus on book edits that felt pointless amidst this profound loss, I decided that maybe this small gesture was one way to thank him and honor him.

So, Mr. Doug, this book is dedicated to you—even though I imagine if you were reading this you would scoff and make a crack about being mentioned in "some nutritionist's book." (Dietitians *hate* being called nutritionists, by the way.)

This book is dedicated to everything you did for your field of sports medicine and athletic training. To everything you did for the field of sports nutrition as you helped me grow my department and advocated for holistic sports medicine services. To everything you did for Purdue. To everything you did for all the athletes you served over the course of your career. And to everything you did for me personally. The void you're leaving will be impossible to fill.

For those of you who have bothered to read this page, I hope too that you'll take a lesson out of Doug's playbook. Show everyone kindness, regardless of their background. Take time to stop and listen to those around you and show them that you care. Work hard, but play (and love on your family) harder. Never take yourself too seriously and stay humble, even amidst substantial success.

I hope they have a rum and Coke poured for you in heaven, Doug. Miss you and Boiler Up.

Contents

PART II: FINE-TUNE YOUR FUELING FOR ANY SCHEDULE

Preface

Welcome! I'm excited that you're here and presumably looking for a way to level up your performance as an athlete. As I often share with the athletes I work with who have reached an elite level, "Congrats! Everyone is good here. How are you going to separate yourself?" It's true that as you progress through the ranks of your sport the competition gets better and better, and the margin that separates good and great becomes smaller and smaller. Although many things contribute to finding yourself on the "great" end of that equation (natural talent, strength training, conditioning, flexibility, skill development, and more), one component of elite performance that should also be considered is nutrition—and more specifically, nutrient timing.

In addition to the fact that you've chosen to hone in on this aspect of your performance, I'm excited that you've chosen to get your information from a qualified source. If you've spent any amount of time on the Internet or social media (or just living on this planet!) you've probably felt like nutrition advice comes from anyone and everyone. Especially as an athlete, you're likely bombarded by advice from current and former coaches, trainers at the gym, teammates and friends, and even people you've never met. The problem, however, is that most people share what they heard from a friend, what they found online, or what worked for them—none of which is backed in science and a lot of which is just plain wrong. This fuels confusion for consumers like you and ultimately leads to a lot of frustration. When working on any aspect of your performance, it's important to put your trust in people who studied and know that field. Just like you wouldn't call a plumber to do your taxes and a quarterback wouldn't call a dietitian to work on his throwing form, you shouldn't call on a strength coach or even a doctor to work on your nutrition.

A registered dietitian (RD)—sometimes called a registered dietitian nutritionist (RDN)—is the only professional who is credentialed to provide individualized nutrition advice. Dietitians have to obtain both a bachelor's degree in nutrition science and a master's degree, complete a yearlong supervised practice, pass an accredited exam, and complete continuing education hours each year to maintain that credential. Furthermore, a board certified specialist in sports dietetics (CSSD) must accumulate 2,000 supervised practice hours in sports nutrition and pass an exam every five years. As an RD and CSSD with over 10 years of experience working with elite-level athletes, I help my athletes lean on recommendations that are based in science, but also take into account their unique likes and dislikes and what is required by their sport and position to be successful.

I recently witnessed this with a group of athletes that worked with me throughout their entire off-season on honing in on different aspects of their nutrition game. Each week was a different subject—eating frequently, including enough carbohydrate, incorporating protein, increasing fruit and veggies, improving their hydration, and even just general self-care with focus on mental health and recovery. The athletes slowly built habits, and toward the end of the off-season were reporting having more energy, seeing better results on the fitness test and in the weight room, and overall feeling better than they had any other year. The coach also happily reported to me that the team could not have had a better off-season, training-wise. While of course other factors likely contributed to this success as well, to think nutrition didn't play a huge part would be naïve. I'm smiling just typing the story!

There are so many aspects of nutrition that can positively affect performance, and athletes can often see big differences in how they feel and perform just by focusing on positively changing one or two habits to start. For some, it may be ensuring they're not skipping meals, or adding healthy, balanced snacks. For others, it may be including enough of a certain macro- or micronutrient or fine-tuning their hydration habits. For those who have a solid handle on their nutrition habits, they might benefit from strategically including certain supplements. One of the most fulfilling parts of my job is when I see changes that an athlete worked on come to fruition and have a direct impact on their performance. Even better is when a whole team does it and you can see all the pieces clicking!

All of these issues and more will be covered in the coming chapters, and you can be assured that everything in this book is backed by science and written with the goal of being practical and easy to implement in your daily routine to ultimately help you be a better athlete. Good luck, and happy fueling!

PART I
Foundations of Effective Fueling

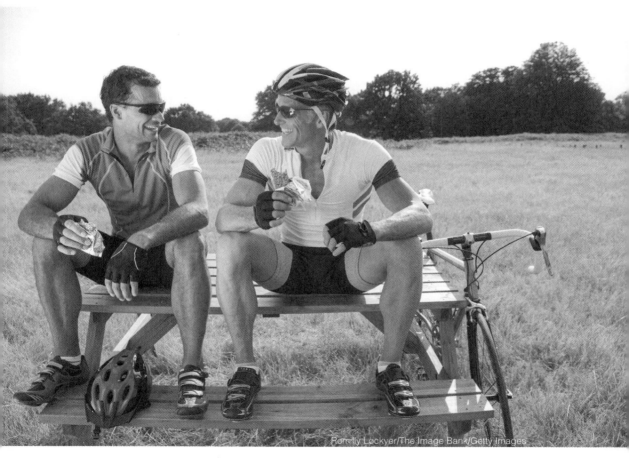

CHAPTER 1

Not *What?* but *When?*: Why Nutrient Timing Matters

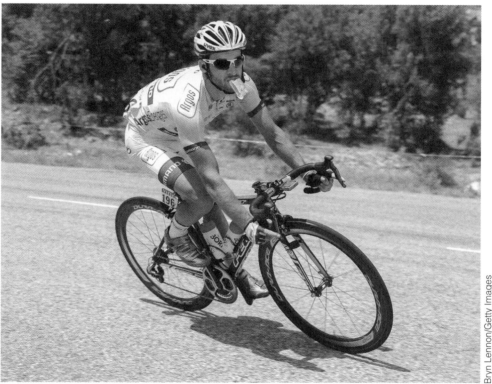

Bryn Lennon/Getty Images

If you've found your way to this book, you may not have to be convinced that what you eat matters. It's likely you already understand that a well-balanced diet influences not just body composition and weight (things that our culture and the media tend to focus on) but also physical and mental health, as well as the risk of various diseases. To take it a step further, if you're reading this book, you probably know that, as an athletic individual, what you eat can also heavily affect your performance. And although the *what* is very important, in many cases the *when* is even more important. Enter nutrient timing, the science of strategically including or excluding specific foods and nutrients from the diet at certain times and in certain amounts to positively influence health and performance.

When athletes set a goal of changing their diet to improve their health and performance, it can sometimes feel overwhelming. Many athletes feel that setting a goal like this means that they need to eat perfectly. This not only leads to stress and anxiety, but it is simply not attainable, even for the most committed athlete—eventually leading to feelings of defeat or failure. Because one of the biggest factors in a successful nutrition plan is sustainability and consistency, I help the athletes I work with reframe this goal: Rather than eat perfectly, eat *purposefully*. Purposeful eating means that you put thought and planning into how you can make your nutrition plan work with your schedule and your training to ensure that you have the resources at hand that you'll need to carry it out. This mindset also allows for life to happen—vacations, parties, and drinks out with friends, as well as obstacles like missing your flight, getting sick, or having especially busy times come up at school or work. If your nutrition plan is too rigid and doesn't allow for your real life to happen, then it's probably not sustainable.

What Does the Research Say?

There is a significant body of research dedicated to the topic of nutrient timing, and like any topic the results vary. However, the vast majority of research on the subject supports the conclusion that proper nutrient timing can pay dividends for health and performance. As mentioned by Arent and colleagues (2020), much of the early work around nutrient timing was centered around the importance of appropriately timed carbohydrate ingestion to support glycogen resynthesis and attenuate glycogen depletion during workouts.

The topic of protein consumption and timing has also sparked much debate in the research world. Although evidence is inconclusive as to whether protein supplementation is truly needed, Willoughby and colleagues (2007) reported greater gains in lean mass and strength with protein supplementation for untrained volunteers following 10 weeks of alternating upper and lower body training four days per week. Early recommendations reference an optimal postworkout anabolic window of 30 minutes to see the most mass gains; however, as research has continued to progress, we now know that this window is bigger than once thought. Although the debate around the exact anabolic window continues, Phillips and Van Loon (2011) conclude that "it is safest to state that athletes who are interested in performance need to consume protein as soon as possible after exercise (S35)." These are just a couple of examples of the research that exists to support the practice of nutrient timing, but the following chapters will dive into many more big picture discussions as well as more nuanced topics.

Putting the Science Into Practice

The ideas of nutrient timing and purposeful eating are especially important when you consider the busy life of an athlete. Whether you're competing at a high school, collegiate, or professional level or competing independently, the training and competition can eat hugely into your schedule. Even for serious athletes without a specific competition schedule, squeezing a workout into your day can be challenging. Because this busy schedule can lead to skipping meals, specific thought might have to be put into the logistics of how food will be consumed—for example, can your choice be eaten on the go? Can you keep it refrigerated? Will you be able to heat it up? Additionally, the effect of training itself sometimes makes it challenging to eat enough, whether as a result of intense training making it hard to meet caloric needs or environmental factors such as heat affecting appetite. For all of these reasons, athletes should consider spending some time planning for their schedules and the challenges that might arise.

Ultimately, the biggest reason to implement nutrient timing strategies into your nutrition plan is simple: the drive to win. It should come

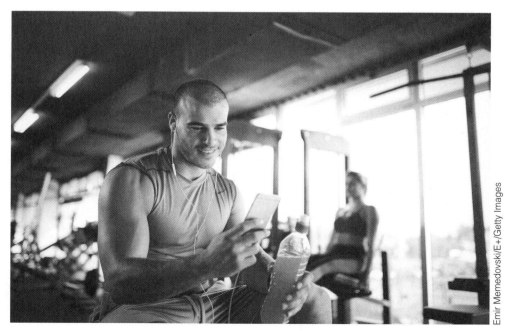

Emir Memedovski/E+/Getty Images

Planning ahead can help meet fueling and hydration goals, even amidst a busy schedule.

as no surprise that many athletes strive to do what they can to improve their chances to set themselves apart. An athlete who is purposeful with what they eat is usually a step ahead of the competition. An athlete who is purposeful with *when* they eat has truly leveled up. Well-constructed nutrient timing can make a big difference by ensuring that the body has adequate nutrients stored and is able to tap into them at the appropriate times. For example, Galloway and colleagues (2014) were able to show that participants who consumed a 6.4 percent carbohydrate beverage 30 minutes prior to exercise lasted over one minute longer until exhaustion compared to participants who consumed the same beverage 120 minutes prior. A layperson might think, "One minute? What's the big deal?"—but an athlete can understand the significance of just one minute when competing! This is especially true at elite levels, where the difference between winning and losing may come down to tenths of a second.

Providing Energy and Fueling Athletic Performance

When you hear the word *energy* your mind might go straight to a cup of coffee or an energy drink. However, though caffeine can provide a quick pick-me-up, it is not a true source of energy. *Energy* refers to the calories used by your body to allow your muscles, organs, and other tissues to function and perform. The foods you eat are stored in different ways so that they can be utilized by the appropriate energy system at the appropriate time.

Depending on the type of activity and the length of time it is performed, the body relies on different nutrients to fuel that performance. If you stood up and sprinted across the room, those few seconds of activity would be fueled by the phosphagen (anaerobic) system, which uses creatine phosphate stored in your muscles to create energy. Creatine phosphate (CP) fuels quick, bursting movements that are crucial to many sports (think sprinting, jumping, diving, hitting, or throwing). If you then kept running out the door and down the street, your body would switch from using the phosphagen system to using the glycolytic (aerobic) system, which uses carbohydrate to fuel performance. This system is used almost exclusively for activities lasting a few minutes— for instance, running or swimming short distances. Imagine if you then kept running to the neighboring town, miles away. As the length of time increased, your body would start utilizing the oxidative system, which is a vital process that uses the micronutrients fat and protein for low- to moderate-intensity exercise that lasts a long time. During a workout your body will seamlessly move in and out of using these different energy systems as long as you have adequately fueled leading up to the event. Figure 1.1 shows the amount and types of energy burned during short-, medium-, and long-duration exercise.

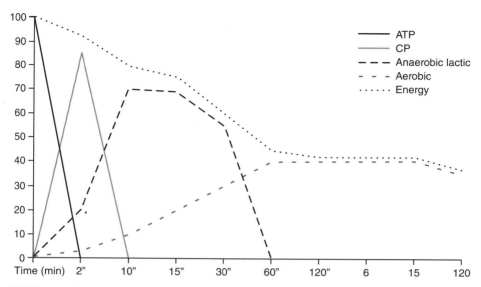

FIGURE 1.1 Relationships between phosphagen and glycolytic energy systems and duration of exercise.

Reprinted by permission from T. Bompa and C.A. Buzzichelli, *Periodization Training for Sports*, 3rd ed. (Champaign, IL: Human Kinetics, 2005), 43.

Building Muscle Mass and Supporting Recovery

Over the course of a day, human skeletal muscle is in a continuous process of both the anabolic process of muscle protein synthesis (MPS), or building new muscle from amino acids, and the catabolic process of muscle protein breakdown (MPB). Collectively these processes are summarized as net muscle protein balance, with the goal that MPS exceeds MPB for a net positive protein balance, supporting overall muscle growth.

Nutrient timing helps minimize the MPB that happens during and after workouts and competition and maximize the MPS that occurs afterwards and generally throughout each day. Tipton, Hamilton, and Gallagher (2018) note that well-timed nutrition can reduce MPB, contributing to a net positive protein balance and ultimately muscle synthesis. Work by Biolo and colleagues (1997) showed that protein immediately after exercise is more anabolic (promotes muscle growth) than protein ingested at other times. Furthermore, it has also been well documented that ingesting carbohydrate and protein together after a workout promotes protein synthesis and a net positive protein balance (Howarth et al. 2009).

Good nutrient timing also helps maximize the carbohydrate that is stored in the liver and muscle tissue in the form of a compound called *glycogen*, the primary fuel source for a majority of activity involved in sport. Having maximum amounts of glycogen available has been shown to delay fatigue and promote overall performance. In their review of glycogen stores and performance, Vigh-Larsen and colleagues (2021) found that adequate glycogen stores are important for high-intensity continuous exercise and that inadequate stores contribute to earlier fatigue. More discussion of glycogen and its function in carbohydrate storage can be found in chapter 3.

Supporting a Healthy Digestive and Immune System

Nutrient timing helps keep your gastrointestinal (GI) system regular, which promotes good overall GI health. Just the act of eating regularly can help movement of digested food through the GI tract, which helps improve absorption of nutrients and water and eliminate waste. Additionally, purposeful nutrient timing helps combat inflammation by providing needed carbohydrate to cells that help control the response to stress. Consistent carbohydrate intake also helps immune cells resist viruses and other threats to immune health—it is literally fueling down to the cellular level. Later chapters will expand on the impact of nutrient timing on inflammation, stress response, and immune health.

Promoting Mental Health and Focus

As will be discussed in much more depth in later chapters, the body's preferred fuel source is carbohydrate, which in its most basic form is glucose, a simple sugar. In fact, the brain prefers to use exclusively glucose. Properly applied nutrient timing strategies keep this energy source consistently available, allowing for improved focus, mental clarity, and decision-making, especially during competition. Conversely, inadequate carbohydrate intake causes blood sugar to dip, which for some people can cause irritability, mood swings, and other unpleasant symptoms. Prolonged inadequate carbohydrate intake can also cause some people to be more prone to anxiety and even depression, though research has not been able to show these effects on a large scale.

Enhancing Recovery

The term *recovery* is used often in sports, often broadly describing the general process of restoring the body to a preexercise state after physical activity. Recovery is a crucial aspect of an athlete's training regimen that involves repairing damaged tissues, replenishing depleted energy stores, and reducing inflammation and muscle soreness—all of which can be influenced by a purposeful approach to nutrition and timing.

Although nutrition is an important component of effective recovery, it is far from the only one.

There are several strategies you can use to support recovery, including getting enough sleep, practicing stress-reducing techniques, and using active recovery techniques such as foam rolling, stretching, or light exercise. Additionally, you should listen to your body and adjust your training and recovery strategies as needed based on your individual needs and goals.

Reducing Risk of Injury

Injury prevention is a product of many factors, including proper warm-up and cool-down, strength training, flexibility, and even some amount of luck. It is therefore unsurprising that there is currently a lack of research to show a direct correlation between nutrient timing and injury prevention. However, as discussed previously, without the appropriate fuel on board you are more likely to lack focus and make poorer decisions, not to mention experience decreased balance and a slower reaction time. All of these can put you at higher risk for injury, as can dehydration, which is another important component of proper nutrient timing (Casa et al. 2000). Although these are acute examples,

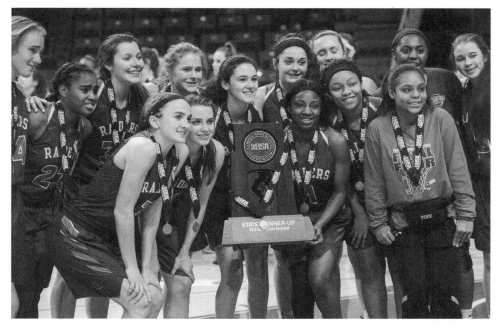

Consistent, purposeful fueling is an important component of seeing success on and off the field of play.

you also can be at higher risk for injury and illness if you are perpetually not promoting good recovery, not getting adequate micronutrients, or not getting enough calories overall. Good recovery practices can help reduce muscle soreness, inflammation, and fatigue, which may all indirectly reduce the risk for injuries by improving physical functioning and reducing risk for overuse injuries.

Hopefully, if you weren't convinced of the need for purposeful fueling when you started reading this chapter, you are now. Regardless of the sport you play or the level at which you play, nutrient timing can play a critical role. For an endurance runner or swimmer, strategic fueling can maximize energy levels and reduce GI distress. For a sprinter or jumper, properly timed fuel intake can promote speed and explosiveness. Even for an athlete playing a skill-based sport, nutrient timing can promote focus, balance, and improved coordination.

The best part? It's science, but it's not rocket science. Many of the principles and practices in this book can be accomplished with whole food sources, on a reasonable budget, and by an athlete at any level. The rest of the book will discuss how you can approach nutrient timing for both the macro- and micronutrients, hydration and supplementation, strategies for different sports and training situations, and some tips on how to navigate that busy schedule and make it all come together. A few examples of athletes will also be highlighted throughout the book to help visualize how these principles can come together for athletes of varying sizes and sports. You can find the one that fits the best and follow along with their story to help conceptualize your unique needs!

CHAPTER 2
Identify Your Timing Needs

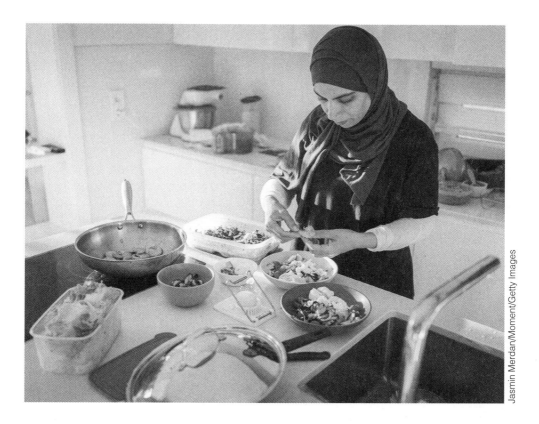

Jasmin Merdan/Moment/Getty Images

One of the most basic nutrient timing questions athletes have is simply, "How often should I be eating?" The answer is much simpler than you might imagine: Regardless of your body size, what sport you participate in, or your weight or performance goals, you should aim to eat a meal or a snack at least every three to four hours. Although some circumstances might warrant eating more often, there is really no reason to eat less frequently. For most people this translates to eating breakfast, lunch, and dinner with a couple of snacks in between. From a practical perspective, eating with this frequency helps curb hunger (not surprisingly, being hungry doesn't promote good physical or mental performance) and can also help athletes meet their caloric needs without feeling

GI discomfort from eating larger, less frequent meals. It also promotes consuming adequate amounts of carbohydrate to support endurance, power, and speed as well as adequate protein to support muscle growth and recovery. Both of these factors will help support positive body composition changes.

Nutrient Timing for Muscle Building and Recovery

Both muscle protein synthesis (MPS) and muscle protein breakdown (MPB) are topics that are of great interest to athletes, and for good reason. If you recall from the last chapter, your body is in a near constant state of these processes, depending on dietary intake of protein and the stimulus that muscle is under. Because muscle mass directly ties to strength, speed, power, and explosiveness, MPS (the ability to build muscle) is important for every single sport. Even sports that aren't traditionally known for requiring large amounts of muscle still rely on qualities like balance, flexibility, and endurance, which are also influenced by muscle mass. Furthermore, any athlete can relate to the desire to avoid injuries, which requires a purposeful and well-designed

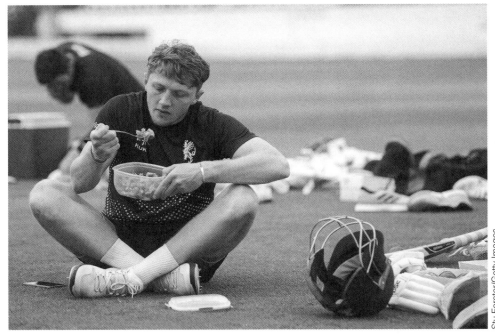

Stu Forster/Getty Images

Sometimes carrying out purposeful nutrient timing requires prepping ahead to ensure you don't miss a fueling opportunity.

What Type of Eater Are You?

Figure 2.1 showcases three different eating patterns and their effects. In the first, which highlights the ideal eating frequency mentioned previously, the athlete never spends too much time in either an energy deficit or energy surplus; rather, energy ebbs and flows as they eat five to six times throughout the day.

The second eating pattern is three big meals, likely eaten five to six hours apart, causing the athlete to spend most of their time in an energy surplus. This scenario comes with the likelihood of the athlete eating past their energy needs and an increased propensity to gain body fat.

The third eating pattern is seen most often in young athletes. The athlete goes a large part of the day without eating anything (perhaps they woke up late and skipped lunch, as so many young athletes do), so that even when they backload calories at night they've now spent most of their day in a caloric deficit. This scenario not only puts the athlete at risk to break down muscle, but ironically makes them more likely to gain body fat as a result of an increased insulin response (discussed later in chapter 8) when they finally eat that late meal. All three scenarios had a similar overall caloric intake across the same 24 hours, but simply by being purposeful with timing, the first eating pattern has positively affected body composition—not to mention has almost certainly been more enjoyable for the athlete.

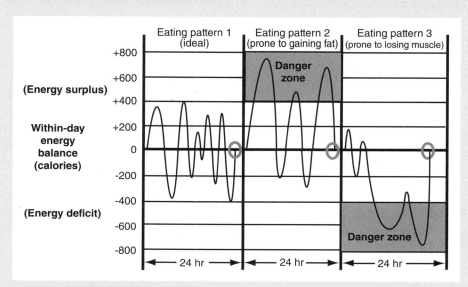

FIGURE 2.1   The same caloric intake across three different eating patterns results in different distributions of energy and can subsequently have different impacts on body composition and performance.

Reprinted by permission from D. Benardot, *Advanced Sports Nutrition*, 3rd ed. (Champaign, IL: Human Kinetics, 2021), 269.

strength and conditioning plan. Most athletes put a considerable amount of time into developing their strength, conditioning, balance, and flexibility, so it makes sense to maximize these efforts through purposeful nutrition.

A common misconception is that MPS happens primarily during a strength and conditioning session, when in fact the opposite is true. During vigorous activity, muscle proteins are actually broken down and damaged, and tiny rips and tears are created in the muscle fibers. Only after the session has concluded does the body start the process of repairing those fibers and working to build new muscle fibers. This process happens all day long and requires the appropriate building blocks (i.e., protein) to do so. The body needs to be in a net positive protein balance to support MPS, meaning it needs more protein available than is being used by other bodily processes. Therefore, one of the quickest ways to hinder this process of recovery and new growth is to not provide those building blocks—in other words, by skipping meals.

Understanding Your Specific Needs

Understanding your energy needs is important, but especially so for athletes. When calculating energy needs it's important to understand the different categories that contribute to your total needs, or total daily energy expenditure (TDEE). These three categories are as follows:

1. *Basal metabolic rate (BMR).* Your BMR is the number of calories that your body needs over the course of 24 hours just to support basic functions at rest, like breathing, digesting food, regulating temperature and pH, and maintaining brain function. Caloric needs are often much higher than what people anticipate, especially for very active individuals. Diets recommending as few as 1,600, 1,200, or even 800 calories per day are commonplace in the media and in certain fitness circles. However, these very low calorie suggestions may not even cover your BMR, let alone your daily activity. A common topic of interest in this area is the long-held belief that metabolism (which can be thought of as similar to BMR) declines steadily with age, beginning as early as age 30 or 40. However, a recent study by Pontzer and colleagues (2021) using a massive cross-sectional study cohort of over 6,400 individuals showed that BMR actually stays relatively stable until after age 60, at which point it begins to decline. The study also found that the decline in BMR was mostly attributed to loss in muscle mass rather than aging itself. With this in mind, it's a

good goal for adults (especially older adults) to maintain as much muscle mass as possible.

2. *Physical activity (PA)*. A large contributor to your total daily energy needs is your physical activity. This includes your workouts as well as activities of daily living like walking. For athletes this number can be quite high and—in some cases—almost equal to BMR. Similar to the effect of aging on BMR, physical activity can decrease over time because it tends to be harder to maintain the same intensity of exercise as you age. It's therefore worth recognizing that the same amount of time spent exercising might not yield the same energy expenditure as you age or even just begin exercising less formally.

3. *Thermic effect of food (TEF)*. TEF refers to the energy expended to digest, absorb, and store the nutrients from the food you've just eaten. Although this number is not significant on its own, it does factor in slightly when understanding your TDEE.

Although calculating your energy needs can be helpful, it's also important to recognize the limitations of such calculations. For one, estimations of your energy needs, caloric expenditure of certain activities, and even caloric content of certain foods are just that—estimations—and they depend on a number of different factors from day to day. It is also important to recognize your own limitations in handling this sort of information. If you have struggled with an eating disorder or disordered eating, or if you have the tendency to become very fixated on numbers, you are probably better off skipping this section and focusing on the more broad recommendations later in this chapter.

Calculating Basal Metabolic Rate

If you do feel like having an estimation of your daily energy needs would be helpful for you, proceed with the following calculations to determine your needs based on your physical activity. There are many equations that can be used to calculate energy needs, which use different anthropometric measures of varying nuance. The Mifflin-St. Jeor (1990) equation will be used here, largely because it is simple and considered one of the more accurate equations used to estimate BMR.

$$\text{Males: } (10 \times \text{weight in kg}) + (6.25 \times \text{height in cm}) - (5 \times \text{age in years}) + 5$$

$$\text{Females: } (10 \times \text{weight in kg}) + (6.25 \times \text{height in cm}) - (5 \times \text{age in years}) - 161$$

Athlete Profiles

Throughout the book we will follow three hypothetical athletes through their daily lives to provide some tangible examples on how to apply the different recommendations that you'll see.

Athlete 1: Jenny

Jenny is 22 years old. She is 5 feet, 6 inches (167.64 cm) tall and weighs 140 pounds (63.50 kg). She plays soccer at the collegiate level.

Athlete 2: Doug

Doug is 45 years old. He is 5 feet, 10 inches (177.8 cm) tall and weighs 165 pounds (74.84 kg). He is an endurance athlete who regularly trains for and participates in marathons and triathlons.

Athlete 3: Thomas

Thomas is 18 years old. He is 6 feet, 4 inches (193.04 cm) tall and weighs 285 pounds (129.27 kg). He is an American football player competing at the collegiate level with hopes of playing professionally.

Using the above equations for the sample athletes, Jenny's BMR would be approximately 1,412 calories per day, Doug's BMR would be approximately 1,640 calories per day, and Thomas's BMR would be approximately 2,414 calories per day. To see how these were calculated, flip to the appendix.

Factoring in Physical Activity

Once you've calculated your BMR, it's important to calculate what your physical activity contributes to your total energy needs. To do so, first decide which of the following activity categories best describes you:

- *Sedentary.* This reflects little or no exercise.
- *Lightly active (light exercise or sports 1-3 days per week).* This might be reflective of off days or weeks or times that activity is very limited due to injury.
- *Moderately active (moderate exercise or sports 3-5 days per week).* This might include lighter training periods when you are not training every day of the week and doing more strength and skill training with minimal conditioning.
- *Very active (hard exercise or sports 6-7 days per week).* This would likely be reflective of normal training for many athletes, during which training is occurring most or all days of the week, for at

least a couple of hours, with a mix of strength and skill training as well as conditioning.

- *Extra active (very hard exercise or sports and physical job or twice daily training).* Examples of this would include athletes who are in a very high training load with heavy conditioning or very high mileage, or athletes who are practicing multiple times per day (including athletes who may be participating in multiple sports at once).

Now, multiply your activity level by your calculated BMR based on the following equations:

$$\text{Sedentary} = \text{BMR} \times 1.2$$

$$\text{Lightly active} = \text{BMR} \times 1.375$$

$$\text{Moderately active} = \text{BMR} \times 1.55$$

$$\text{Very active} = \text{BMR} \times 1.725$$

$$\text{Extra active} = \text{BMR} \times 1.9$$

Calculating Thermic Effect of Food

To calculate an estimate of your thermic effect of food, multiply your BMR by 0.1. Add this to the number you just calculated for your physical activity.

With these three categories in mind, total daily energy expenditure (TDEE) for Jenny, Doug, and Thomas could be estimated as the following:

Jenny: 2,677 calories

Doug: 3,428 calories

Thomas: 4,116 calories

As mentioned, knowing their TDEE can be helpful for some, but for many people a less structured approach works just as well or even better. This is especially true for people who tend to get obsessive over calories eaten, calories burned, and their intake and activity in general. Obsession over these kinds of numbers can quickly lead to disordered eating tendencies, which are incredibly detrimental to health and performance. It also tends to be unrealistic to be extremely structured with these numbers, because life often doesn't cooperate: It's hard (and usually stressful) to try to plan for every single possibility when it comes to food and schedule. I often encourage athletes to approach their daily needs by focusing on eating every three to four hours, and by trying to balance their plate with carbohydrate, protein, and fruits and vegetables. Of course, *which* carbohydrates and proteins you choose are important, as is how your foods are prepared, but the simple habit of approaching your meals and snacks with this balanced outlook can go a long way toward promoting great habits without making you feeling stressed in the name of calories in and calories out.

Supporting Performance With Macronutrients

As you determine what your individual nutritional needs might be, it's best to start from a broad perspective and work on getting more specific. You may have grown up learning about food groups like grains, meat, dairy, fruits, and vegetables and how those fit into the food pyramid—or more recently, into MyPlate. In the world of sports nutrition, discussion is usually centered around the three macronutrients: carbohydrate, protein, and fat. Every single thing that you eat or drink (with the exception of water and alcohol) comprise carbohydrate, protein, and fat. Each macronutrient is important and serves many different purposes in the body and in supporting performance. Each macronutrient will be discussed in depth in the following chapters, but the following sections will provide a quick overview of carbohydrate, protein, and fat.

Eat for Energy With Carbohydrate

Carbohydrate, quite simply, provides energy. In fact, it is the primary fuel source for most activity. As mentioned in chapter 1, carbohydrate in its most simple form, glucose, is the preferred source of fuel for the brain. I often encourage athletes to think of their body as a car and carbohydrate as the gasoline. Any activity that you do burns through some of this fuel tank, and how quickly that happens depends on the type of exercise you're doing as well as the intensity and duration.

Foods rich in carbohydrate include grains like bread, rice, pasta, and cereals, along with fruits and vegetables—especially starchy vegetables like potatoes, corn, and peas. An often overlooked source of carbohydrate is dairy products like milk and yogurt, which contain a specific type of carbohydrate called lactose. Carbohydrate is a frequent target of criticism, and it is wildly common to see diet suggestions that revolve around limiting or cutting carbohydrate out of your diet. Although doing so promotes temporary weight loss, it is just that—temporary. Carbohydrate needs are discussed in detail in chapter 3, but for now, suffice to say that carbohydrate is a vital part of anyone's diet, especially an athlete.

Build and Repair With Protein

Protein is vital for many biological processes. Although the most notable might be acting as the material for building and repairing cells, it's also involved in enzymatic reactions, hormone and pH regulation, immunity, and digestion. Foods rich in protein include meat; poultry; fish; shellfish; eggs; dairy products like milk, cheese, and cottage cheese; and some plant-based sources like beans and legumes. Protein is often considered the most important macronutrient in the sport and fitness realm, and though athletic populations do have higher protein needs than the general public, protein should be approached with balance and consistency just like carbohydrate.

Fuel With Healthy Fats

The third macronutrient, fat, is usually viewed in a negative light. However, fat also plays an essential role in health. Maintaining a healthy amount of body fat is necessary to protect internal organs and maintain healthy hormone activity. Additionally, fat in the diet also serves important functions, most notably in helping the digestive system absorb fat-soluble vitamins. That said, it is still important to not overdo it on total fat intake and to make sure that you're limiting unhealthy fats (trans fats and hydrogenated oils) and including plenty of healthy fats (monounsaturated and polyunsaturated fatty acids). The different types and sources of fat will be discussed in chapter 5.

Building a Balanced Plate

So how do these macronutrients translate to something practical? It may surprise you, but you don't need to count your macros to have a purposeful approach to balancing your plate. A much simpler and less stressful way to start approaching this idea of balance is to think about dedicating certain proportions of your plate to the different macronutrients.

A good baseline plate has one-third dedicated to carbohydrate, one-third dedicated to protein, and one-third dedicated to fruits and vegetables. You'll notice that I won't mention dedicating part of your plate to fat at any point: Even though a certain amount of fat is necessary, fat tends to find its way into our diets via many different foods and does not often need purposeful addition. Instead, the third category is fruits and vegetables. Although fruits and vegetables are generally carb-rich,

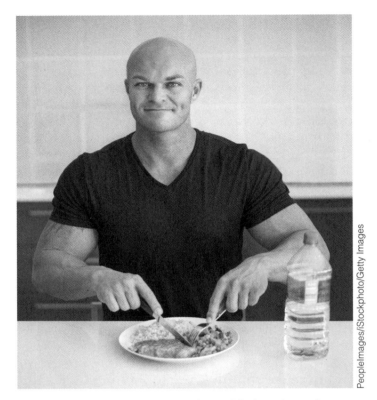

Peoplelmages/iStockphoto/Getty Images

Balance your plate with carbohydrates, protein, and fruit and veggies to ensure you're meeting all of your needs.

they are not very energy-dense. This means that most of them don't contain the same concentration of calories per serving as other sources of carbohydrates like grains. Fruits and veggies also contain the vast majority of the vitamins, minerals, and fiber in our diets. For these reasons, making a concerted effort to consistently get them on your plate alongside grains is key.

There are also some foods that might throw you for a loop upon first glance. A handful of vegetables, such as corn, potatoes, and peas, are more carbohydrate rich than most so we tend to categorize them as carbohydrates. Some foods, such as milk, yogurt, beans and lentils, also pull double duty and are rich in both carbohydrate and protein. These double hitters fall into either category, making them versatile depending on the meal.

The baseline plate depicted in figure 2.2 is a nice starting point for many athletes because it ensures adequate carbohydrate to fuel activity and training, adequate protein to support MPS, and plenty of fruits and veggies to provide necessary vitamins, minerals, and fiber. If you

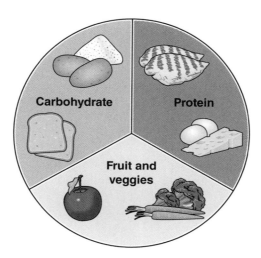

FIGURE 2.2   Example plate showing equal thirds of carbohydrate, protein, and fruit and veggies.

Reprinted by permission from L. Link, *The Healthy Former Athlete* (New York: Skyhorse Publishing, 2018).

are eating every three to four hours and ensuring that your plate has this balanced approach, you should feel good about the foundation that you're laying for the rest of your fueling.

Of course, individual needs, training situations, and goals will influence this baseline plate. For example, higher carbohydrate intake would be warranted for athletes in endurance-based sports (e.g., soccer, triathlon, long-distance running, cycling, skiing, swimming), periods of intense training (multiple sessions per day, preseason training camp, heavy conditioning, etc.), and athletes participating in multiple sports, which is especially common in high school. This example plate would be closer to one-half carbohydrate, one-fourth protein, and one-fourth fruits and vegetables (figure 2.3).

Other situations might warrant an opposite approach—decreasing carbohydrate and protein closer to one-fourth and increasing fruits and vegetables closer to one-half (figure 2.4). This approach would be warranted for athletes in lower-expenditure or skill-based sports (excluding high workload time frames like conditioning). Sports that fit in this category might include diving, bowling, baseball or softball, archery, or rifle. It also could be appropriate if you are in an off-season, a period of very light training, or are trying to decrease body weight.

One thing I like about this approach is that it never suggests getting rid of any of the three components. It is common to hear nutrition suggestions centered around excluding groups of food or even entire macronutrients. Although this topic could be a book in itself, I'll quickly

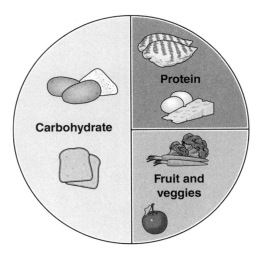

FIGURE 2.3   Example plate showing one-half carbohydrate, one-fourth protein, and one-fourth fruit and veggies.

Reprinted by permission from L. Link, *The Healthy Former Athlete* (New York: Skyhorse Publishing, 2018).

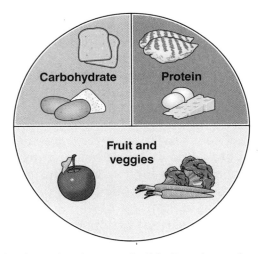

FIGURE 2.4   Example plate showing one-half fruit and veggies, one-fourth carbohydrate, and one-fourth protein.

Reprinted by permission from L. Link, *The Healthy Former Athlete* (New York: Skyhorse Publishing, 2018).

summarize by saying that those approaches are generally not sustainable long term, often lead to short-term weight loss but long-term weight gain, and don't promote good performance. For that reason, any nutrition approach should be sustainable and always include a balance of carbohydrate, protein, and fruits and vegetables.

Making Small, Sustainable Changes

As you think through how you want to approach your diet, I would encourage you to start first with the big picture considerations and focus on only one or two changes at a time. It can be tempting when working on your nutrition habits to immediately try to hone in on getting specific nutrients or start using a certain supplement. However, it's important to make sure your foundational nutrition is in line first. If you have good foundational habits, then you can work on getting more specific.

As an example, first you might evaluate if you are eating frequently enough. Are you currently skipping any meals or snacks that you could work on ensuring you eat? From there, evaluate if your plate is balanced with the three groups discussed previously. Once these foundational measures are in place you can focus on getting the appropriate amounts and types of nutrients.

Even if you want to get more specific with your calorie or macronutrient goals, I would encourage you to start by tracking a few meals over one or two days to get a feel for how you might meet those goals rather than beginning with intensive tracking of every meal every day. The most realistic way for most people to track their intake is by using a meal or calorie tracking app like MyFitnessPal. Even the most sophisticated apps can only provide a general estimate of your intake, so it's important to not get too caught up in minute details. However, this general tracking can be a nice way to help you quantify some of your current habits without getting too caught up in specific numbers.

Remember too that, despite what social media would have you believe at times, changes to your nutrition plan do not have to be—and generally should not be—radical changes. They should be small, sustainable changes that you can be consistent with and build on over time.

Without a solid groundwork, the more specific suggestions and strategies discussed in the coming chapters will be difficult to build on and will be harder for you to carry out. The recommendations in this chapter will therefore help you create a solid nutritional foundation as you dive into more specific macronutrient needs and considerations in the next few chapters.

CHAPTER 3
Go Harder for Longer With Carbohydrates

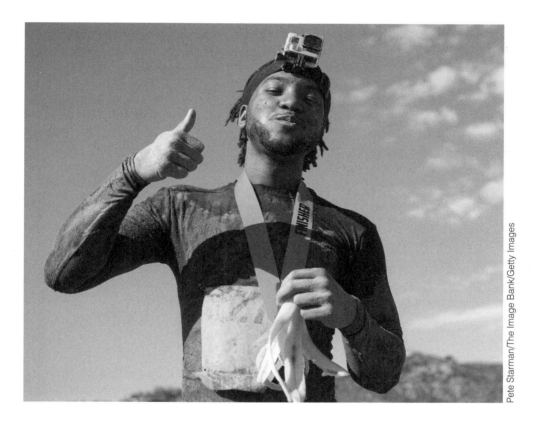

Pete Starman/The Image Bank/Getty Images

As discussed previously, the primary role of carbohydrate is to provide cells with energy. Carbohydrates are organic compounds consisting of sugars, starch, and different types of fiber. For every gram of carbohydrate utilized, the body receives 4 calories in return. When carbohydrate is consumed, it is digested and broken down into simple sugars. Although some may get used right away, most get stored as glycogen, a compound made by combining those sugars with water, which is then deposited in the skeletal muscle and liver. A little bit of the sugar also remains in the bloodstream as blood glucose (commonly known

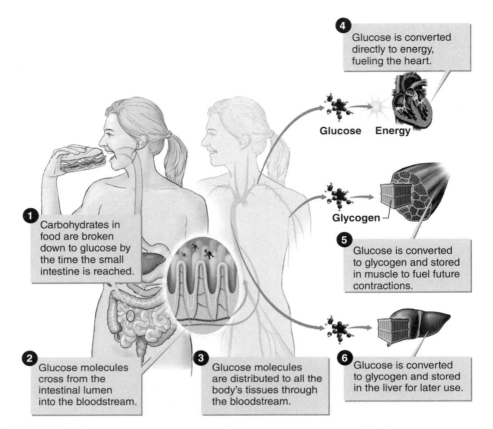

FIGURE 3.1 Carbohydrates are digested and transported within the body to provide fuel for activity.

Reprinted by permission from B. Sharkey, *Fitness Illustrated* (Champaign, IL: Human Kinetics, 2010), 200.

as *blood sugar*) (figure 3.1). When the body breaks down carbohydrate and causes blood sugar to rise, the pancreas produces a hormone called *insulin*, which prompts cells to absorb that blood sugar to either be stored or used as energy. As is the case with any excess macronutrient, the extra carbohydrate will be stored as fat in the body. This concept is often misconstrued, fueling the misconception that carbohydrates are "fattening." It's important to remember that calories from any source can lead to weight gain when consistently consumed in excess, and just like protein synthesis and breakdown are in a constant state of flux, so too are carbohydrate synthesis and breakdown.

Types and Sources of Carbohydrate

As discussed in chapter 1, the simple act of consistently having carbohydrate present in your body can help avoid large swings in blood sugar, which keeps your energy levels steady and helps keep you feeling good throughout the day. Although this is a great starting point for your general health, there are additional considerations to help you optimize your performance as an athlete. The first is the type of carbohydrate that you choose. There are two categories of carbohydrate: simple and complex. Simple carbohydrates tend to be broken down quickly by the digestive system and often cause blood glucose to rise (and subsequently fall) quickly. Complex carbohydrates tend to be digested more slowly and therefore provide more sustained energy rather than causing a spike in blood glucose. Complex carbohydrates, found in whole grains, vegetables, and fruit with the skin on, are a great choice at mealtimes when you have at least an hour or two before your next workout or competition. They can help promote fullness and sustained energy, as well as provide a consistent source of fiber and certain micronutrients in your diet. Note, however, that complex carbohydrates are not an ideal choice if you're heading to do physical activity: Fiber can slow down digestion and can cause bloating, gas, and GI distress when eaten too closely to physical activity.

On the other hand, simple carbohydrates are a fantastic choice for a preworkout time frame. Foods high in simple carbohydrates tend to be refined or "white" grains, fruit without the skin, and even foods high in processed sugar like candy. These foods can certainly be included in mealtimes, but ideally with less frequency than complex carbohydrates.

The Glycemic Index

When it comes to quantifying where a food falls on the simple versus complex carbohydrate scale, there is a measurement system called the glycemic index. Glycemic index is a numerical ranking system that rates carbohydrate based on how quickly it raises blood sugar levels after consumption compared to glucose. Foods with a high glycemic index are rapidly digested and absorbed, leading to a quick and large increase in blood sugar levels, whereas foods with a low glycemic index are more slowly digested and absorbed, resulting in a slower and smaller rise in blood sugar levels. Relative to athletic activities, high glycemic–index foods tend to be simple carbohydrate, great for during and immediately around activity, whereas low glycemic–index foods tend to be more complex carbohydrate that might not sit as well right before activity, but are great for meals and other less active times of the day.

However, they are perfect for including just before and even during workouts or competition. Their simple structure makes them easy to digest, meaning that the body can quickly break them down and get that fuel to the muscles. This quick digestion also tends to mean less GI discomfort, which is a win. Preworkout (less than 60 minutes prior) and intraworkout fueling should include very little to no protein and fat and comprise mostly simple carbohydrate.

Some great sources of easily digested simple carbohydrate include white bread, applesauce, fruit, sports drinks, sports chews or gels, honey, jam, granola bars, and fruit snacks. Table 3.1 provides a more complete reference for foods that are rich in both simple and complex carbohydrate.

TABLE 3.1   Carbohydrate-Rich Foods

Type of carbohydrate		Serving size	Amount of carbohydrate per serving (g)
Simple	Complex		
PASTA AND GRAINS			
Spaghetti		1 cup	43
	Whole-wheat pasta	1 cup	37
White rice		1 cup, cooked	41
	Brown rice	1 cup, cooked	45
Spanish rice		1 cup, cooked	41
	Wild rice	1 cup, cooked	35
	Quinoa	1 cup, cooked	40
	Couscous	1 cup, cooked	37
HOT CEREALS			
Cream of Wheat		1 cup, cooked	21
	Oatmeal	1 cup, cooked	27
	Steel cut oats	1 cup, cooked	28
	Grits	1 cup, cooked	23
COLD CEREALS			
Honey Nut Cheerios		1 cup	25
	Kashi Go Lean	1 cup	35
Frosted Flakes		1 cup	28
Rice Krispies		1 cup	25
	Total	1 cup	23
	Frosted Mini Wheats	1 cup	41
Froot Loops		1 cup	26
	Cheerios	1 cup	22

Type of carbohydrate		Serving size	Amount of carbohydrate per serving (g)
Simple	Complex		
STARCHY VEGETABLES			
Mashed potatoes (no skin)		1 cup	35
	Baked potato	1 cup	37
	Corn	1 cup	41
	Sweet potato	1 cup	41
	Squash	1 cup	22
	Peas	1 cup	25
	Split pea soup	1 cup	35
	Beans or lentils	1 cup	45
BREAD AND BAKED GOODS			
White bread		1 slice	13
	Whole-wheat bread	1 slice	17
Plain bagel		1 bagel	52
	Whole-wheat bagel	1 bagel	61
English muffin		1 muffin	25
Dinner roll		1 small roll	15
Corn bread		1 2-inch square	20
Pita bread		1 6-inch round	33
Hot dog or hamburger bun		1 bun	22
	Corn tortilla	1 small	11
Flour tortilla		1 6-inch round	15
Biscuit		1 biscuit	17
Pancakes		1 4-inch round	11
Waffles		1 7-inch round	25
Muffin		1 medium	65
SNACKS, CRACKERS, BARS			
Saltine crackers		6 crackers	13
	Whole-grain crackers	6 crackers	14
	Chewy granola bar with oats	1 bar	17
	Clif bar	1 bar	43
Pretzels		15 pretzels	25
Rice cakes		2 cakes	14

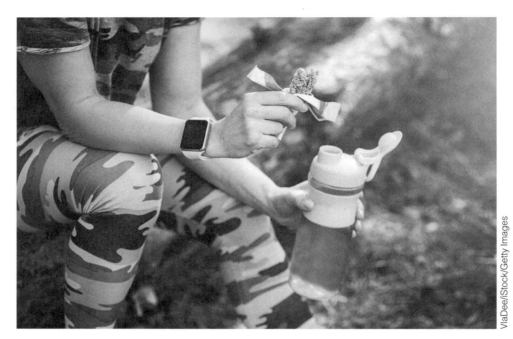

ViaDee/iStock/Getty Images

Quick-digesting carbohydrates consumed just before and during activity help promote improved performance.

In summary, both simple and complex carbohydrates have a purpose and play a role in your day-to-day diet. Jeukendrup (2010) highlights this concept by emphasizing that quickly digested carbohydrate can be beneficial for athletes during exercise when fast-acting energy is needed. However, he also notes that consuming too much simple carbohydrate can lead to blood sugar spikes and crashes, which can negatively affect performance. In addition to using the recommended amounts found later in the chapter, it is advised that you trial your competition fueling plan during practice to see how it affects your performance.

Carbohydrate Needs for Athletes

Now that you have an understanding of what foods contain carbohydrates and what kind of carbohydrates might work best in certain situations, let's talk about how much you need as an athlete. I often share with athletes that the quickest way to negatively affect their performance (outside of dehydration) is to not eat enough carbohydrate. It is well documented that appropriate carbohydrate intake supports performance. Unfortunately, one of the most common misconceptions among athletes is a vast underestimation of the amount of carbohydrate elite-level athletes need. Female athletes, particularly endurance athletes, are especially unlikely to achieve the recommended carbohydrate intake (Burke et al. 2001). This is likely a result of periodic or chronic restriction of total energy intake in order to achieve or maintain low levels of body fat. With how much misinformation about carbohydrate is perpetuated by the media, it's no wonder that this is so common. We are constantly exposed to claims that carbohydrates are "bad," "fattening," and sometimes even "toxic" or "poison." However, these claims are false and exist only to use fearmongering as a tactic to sell you the latest book, fad diet, supplement, or meal replacement. The reality is that humans need carbohydrate, and for athletes this macronutrient is even more important and needed in higher amounts.

Coyle and colleagues (1986) were some of the first to show the importance of carbohydrate to athletic performance, with the finding that cyclists who consumed a carbohydrate-rich drink during exercise were able to maintain a higher power output and delay fatigue compared to those who consumed the placebo. Notably, they showed that this delay in onset of fatigue is attributable to a maintenance in blood glucose concentration, not just a slowing of glycogen depletion. A more recent review by Nédélec and colleagues (2015) shows that the research continues to support these findings.

Jentjens and Jeukendrup (2003) showed carbohydrate intake to be important after exercise as well. Because glycogen depletion in the muscles and liver is a major cause of fatigue during prolonged exercise, they suggested that the rate of glycogen resynthesis during recovery can be enhanced by consuming carbohydrate immediately after exercise. In one study cited by the authors, cyclists who consumed a carbohydrate drink immediately after exercise were able to achieve higher rates of glycogen resynthesis and to perform better in subsequent exercise tests compared to those who did not consume a carbohydrate drink. It was also found that a low-carbohydrate diet led to a decrease in muscle glycogen stores and a decrease in endurance capacity in trained athletes. Conversely, a high-carbohydrate diet led to an increase in muscle glycogen stores and an increase in endurance capacity: A review by Haff et al. (2003) noted that carbohydrate intake can enhance strength and power production during resistance training by providing a readily available source of fuel for the muscles. It was particularly noted that daily maintenance of glycogen levels was likely crucial for maximizing gains in both conditioning and resistance training. The authors additionally noted that athletes engaging in anaerobic training may benefit from a carbohydrate supplement's ability to decrease stress on the immune system.

Figure 3.2 shows what percentage of each activity is fueled by the different macronutrients and provides an excellent example of how much carbohydrate is needed to fuel activity. As you can see, the only activity that relies heavily on fat as a substrate for fuel is rest and light to moderate activity, with both still requiring a fair amount of carbohydrate

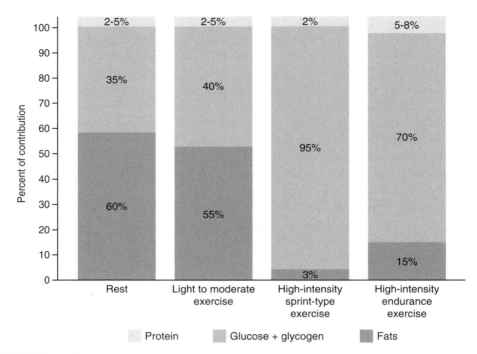

FIGURE 3.2   The contribution of the macronutrients protein (light gray), carbohydrate (medium gray), and fat (dark gray) to energy metabolism at rest and during various intensities of exercise.

Adapted by permission from W.D. McArdle, F.I. Katch, and V.L. Katch, *Sports and Exercise Nutrition*, 5th ed. (Philadelphia, PA: Wolters Kluwer, 2018).

in the form of glucose and glycogen. When you look at high-intensity sprint-type exercise and high-intensity endurance exercise, both rely heavily on carbohydrate, sprint-type exercise almost exclusively so. What is important for athletes to remember is that those last two categories describe most sports (with the exception of some skill-based sports). Between sprint-type exercises like jumping, sprinting, hitting, diving, and other explosive movements, and endurance-based exercises like running, swimming, and rowing, most sports involve some combination of these activities.

How much carbohydrate you need over the course of an entire day correlates with how much energy you have expended that day. You need a certain baseline amount every day to help fuel basic bodily functions—most notably, brain function. Beyond that baseline amount, your carbohydrate needs will depend on the type and amount of activity that you are participating in. This is similar to factoring physical activity into your energy needs, as discussed in chapter 2, but geared specifically toward carbohydrate needs. Recommendations are shown in table 3.2 and in the appendix.

TABLE 3.2 Carbohydrate Recommendations Based on Exercise Intensity and Volume

Type of activity	Example situations	Recommended carbohydrate intake (g/kg)
Very light (low-intensity or skill-based) training, or moderate training <60 min/day	• Off-season training • Skill-based sports with very little conditioning or endurance requirements (e.g., golf, bowling, diving) • Athletes trying to reduce body weight	3-5
Moderate-intensity training, 60 min/day	• Light training periods • Sports with low endurance needs (e.g., baseball, softball, field or short-distance events in track and swimming)	5-7
Moderate- to high-intensity endurance training, 1-3 hr/day	• High training periods • Combo sports (e.g., basketball, tennis, volleyball) • Endurance sports (e.g., running, cycling, swimming, soccer, lacrosse)	6-10
Moderate- to high-intensity endurance training, 4-5 hr/day	• Athletes with multiple endurance-based practices a day • Athletes competing in multiple sports simultaneously • Ultraendurance training with very high mileage	8-12

Adapted by permission from E. Rosenbloom and J. Coleman, *Sports Nutrition: A Practice Manual for Professionals*, 5th ed., edited by C. Karpinski and C.A. Rosenbloom (Chicago: Academy of Nutrition and Dietetics, 2012).

Carbohydrate Timing

Although meeting your total carbohydrate goal is important, the timing of when you eat it, how much you eat, and which kind you choose for certain situations is key to athletic success.

Before the Workout

The hours leading up to activity are arguably the most important time frame for being intentional about carbohydrate intake. As mentioned, it often surprises athletes how much carbohydrate is needed to support activity, especially when that activity is very long (over two hours) or

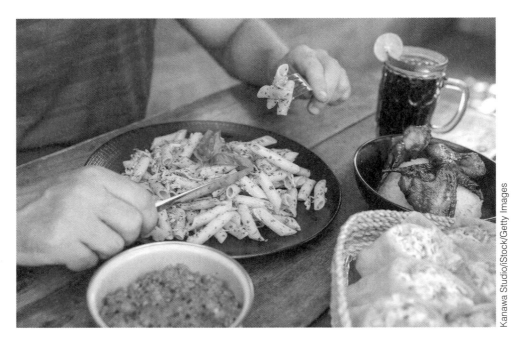

Include a variety of carbohydrate-rich foods like pasta, rice, bread, and other grains to help meet total carbohydrate needs.

involves a lot of aerobic, endurance-based activity. As mentioned earlier, I often use the analogy that your body is like a car, and carbohydrate is like the gasoline. If you were leaving for a road trip, you would likely stop and fill up your tank before you got on the highway. You can think about preworkout fueling in a similar sense. You want to top off your "fuel tank" (carbohydrate stored as glycogen) before you start the workout. This can help prevent hunger during a prolonged workout and provide glucose to your brain, which can help improve cognitive function.

An easy way to remember how much carbohydrate you need before a workout (and how much your stomach can realistically digest) is the "4, 3, 2, 1" rule (table 3.3). If the planned activity is four hours away, you

TABLE 3.3   Carbohydrate Timing Recommendations

Time before exercise	Carbohydrate recommendation
1 hour	1 g/kg
2 hours	2 g/kg
3 hours	3 g/kg
4 hours	4 g/kg

should aim for 4 grams of carbohydrate per kilogram of body weight; if the planned activity is three hours away, you need 3 grams per kilogram, and so forth. This is not to imply that you should eat this much carbohydrate at each of these intervals—that would be far more than you need. This is simply to help guide you on how much you should aim for depending on the time frame leading up to activity.

On the higher end of that range (i.e., three to four hours away from activity), this might look more like a meal. At this time you can usually be a little more liberal with which kind of carbohydrate you choose because you will have ample time to digest and still feel at your best while performing. As you get closer to one to two hours before activity, not only do you need to adjust your carbohydrate intake accordingly (think more like a snack), but you need to be increasingly conscious of what kind of carbohydrate you're eating. At this point you'll want to choose simple carbohydrate instead of complex, which takes longer to digest, and if you are one hour or less from activity, I recommend limiting protein and fat completely. (As a reminder, good sources of simple carbohydrate can be found in table 3.1.) This will make quickly delivered carbohydrate fuel available for your muscles and allow less potential for GI distress. Once you start activity, your body must increase blood flow to your muscles and away from your GI tract, which can lead to decreased performance—no one performs at their best when they feel nauseous and weighed down by undigested food in their stomach! If you are ever between time frames (e.g., 3.5 hr from activity) I would recommend rounding down to the lower amount; you will still be getting a good amount of carbohydrate without running the risk of feeling too full.

If you struggle to eat much before a morning workout, you should aim to have at least a small amount (around 30 g) of carbohydrate before your workout to help improve performance and delay fatigue. If you are preparing for a short (<60 min) or very light workout that will require minimal exertion (light jog-through, stretching, etc.) you are likely fine to not consume a preworkout carbohydrate. If you are doing a good job of eating frequently (as discussed in chapter 2), then you should have consumed a meal in the few hours leading up to activity, which should be adequate to fuel a low-intensity or very short workout.

Ensure that whatever you choose for your preworkout meal or snack is something that you have tested beforehand, especially if it's a competition day. You should choose foods that are familiar to you and that you know won't cause GI upset. Testing different approaches and foods during training can help you fine-tune a plan that works well for you so that you're prepared for competition. Competition fueling will be discussed further in chapters 10 and 11.

Case Studies

Let's now revisit our examples of athletes from chapter 2.

Jenny

If Jenny were having a pregame meal three-and-a-half hours prior to a soccer game, she would aim to have around 190 grams of carbohydrate. It might look something like the following (CHO = abbreviation for carbohydrate):

Breakfast

   2 cups of cooked oatmeal (made with milk) (85 g CHO)

   1 medium banana (27 g CHO)

   1/4 cup of raisins (35 g CHO)

   1 piece of toast with peanut butter (30 g CHO)

Doug

If Doug were eating three hours prior to a training run, he should aim for about 225 grams of carbohydrate. His meal might look like the following:

Lunch

   Sandwich on whole-wheat bread with turkey and cheese (40 g CHO)

   1 individual bag pretzels (22 g CHO)

   1 cup of yogurt (45 g CHO) mixed with 1/2 cup of granola (32 g CHO)

   1 large apple (34 g)

   20 fl oz sports drink (36 g CHO)

Thomas

If Thomas had a late night game and planned to eat his pregame meal three-and-a-half hours before kickoff, he could aim for up to 390 grams of carbohydrate. If this amount felt difficult to obtain, he could consider having some of this via the meal and another smaller snack closer to game time:

Dinner

   3 cups of cooked pasta (129 g CHO)

   1.5 cups of tomato sauce (23 g CHO)

   4 oz of cooked ground turkey (0 g CHO)

   1 cup of cooked broccoli (6 g CHO)

   2 breadsticks (40 g CHO)

   1/2 cup of sliced carrots (6 g CHO)

   20 fl oz sports drink (36 g CHO)

Snack (1 hour prior)

2 peanut butter and jelly sandwiches (80 g CHO)

1 individual bag of goldfish (20 g CHO)

20 fl oz sports drink (36 g CHO)

Remember to flip to the appendix for a detailed breakdown on how recommendations for Jenny, Doug, and Thomas were calculated!

During the Workout

Depending on the intensity and duration of your workout or competition, having intraworkout carbohydrate may or may not be necessary. If you do include intraworkout carbohydrate, ensure that it is a simple carbohydrate—it should be as easy and quick as possible to digest. Ideal intraworkout snacks are carb-rich and easy to eat or drink quickly, especially if you don't have long to get it down. Great examples include sports drinks, gels, or chews, as well as similar products like fruit snacks and even chewy or gummy candy. However, if you do choose these options,

Intraworkout Carbohydrate Recommendations

- For workouts lasting 30 minutes or less, supplementing carbohydrate during the workout is unnecessary, and proper preworkout fueling should be more than enough.
- For high-intensity workouts lasting 30 to 60 minutes, it may be beneficial to supplement small amounts of carbohydrate during the workout or competition. This could be as simple as sipping a sports drink a few times during the workout.
- For high-intensity endurance and intermittent exercise lasting one to two hours, a good rule of thumb is to have 30 grams of carbohydrate per hour during the workout; for endurance exercise lasting two to three hours you should aim to have 60 grams per hour. In these cases, this could look like having a sports drink and a simple carbohydrate at halftime of a game or at a break during a long, strenuous practice.
- For endurance and ultraendurance exercise lasting three hours or more, it is recommended to have up to 90 grams of carbohydrate per hour and try to include multiple forms of carbohydrate (like glucose and fructose) to increase the body's ability to absorb the carbohydrate efficiently enough to keep up with this high workload.

it is vital to ensure proper hydration, because these highly concentrated carb-rich foods and drinks can reduce how much fluid is absorbed and put you at risk for an upset stomach and dehydration.

Kerksick and colleagues (2017) noted that high-intensity exercise specifically requires aggressive carbohydrate and fluid replacement, especially if conditions are hot or humid. Consumption of 1.5 to 2 cups (12-16 fl oz) of a 6 to 8 percent carbohydrate solution (6-8 g carbohydrate per 100 mL of fluid) has been shown as an effective strategy to replace fluid, sustain blood glucose levels, and promote performance.

It can be challenging to ingest higher amounts of carbohydrate because of the limiting rate at which the gut can digest carbohydrate. Even its simplest form, glucose, can only be absorbed at about 1 gram per kilogram per minute. With this in mind, a helpful strategy in ultraendurance settings is to combine simple sugars. For example, combining glucose and fructose (another simple sugar often found in fruits) allows you to almost double that utilization rate to 1.8 grams of carbohydrate per kilogram per minute. Examples of foods that combine glucose and fructose are white table sugar, agave nectar, and maple syrup. Types of simple sugars are listed in table 3.4.

These recommendations are for well-trained athletes. If you are a more casual exerciser or perform at lower overall intensities, you may

TABLE 3.4   Types of Simple Sugars

Name	Description	Source
Glucose	Most common simple sugar and the primary source of energy for the body	Many foods, including fruits, vegetables, and grains
Fructose	Used as a sweetener in processed foods; can cause GI upset if too much is consumed at once, especially before workouts	Fruits, vegetables, and honey
Galactose	Structurally similar to glucose, with a similar level of sweetness	Dairy products
Sucrose	Disaccharide made up of glucose and fructose; commonly known as table sugar	Many foods, including candy, baked goods, and soft drinks
Lactose	Disaccharide made up of glucose and galactose	Milk and dairy products
Maltose	Disaccharide made up of two glucose molecules	Commonly found in beer and malted drinks

not digest and utilize carbohydrate as quickly and may need to start with lower amounts if you experience GI distress.

After the Workout

The time that follows the completion of a workout is incredibly important for recovery. Many athletes have heard about the importance of protein after finishing a workout (discussed in chapter 4), but many underestimate the importance of carbohydrate in this time frame. A workout lasting two to three hours can largely deplete your body's fuel tank (stored glycogen), and it's important to start replenishing this stored fuel right away—ideally within 30 to 45 minutes of finishing a workout. Although waiting longer won't completely negate the benefits, the body is most efficient at repairing muscle tissue and restoring glycogen levels during this time frame. This can be attributed to increased blood flow to muscles after exercise and muscle cells that are more likely to take up available glucose as a result of heightened insulin sensitivity. Research backs this up: Aragon and Schoenfield (2013) concluded that glycogen resynthesis is most rapid in the first few hours after exercise, and that consuming carbohydrate during this time can help maximize glycogen synthesis. Similarly, Ivy and colleagues (1985) showed that delaying carbohydrate ingestion after exercise reduces the rate of muscle glycogen storage.

It is recommended to consume 1 to 1.2 grams of carbohydrate per kilogram of body weight per hour for the first four hours following exercise. Breaking this into small amounts of carbohydrate more frequently (every 15-30 min) may especially enhance this process, as can including high glycemic–index foods (described earlier in the chapter). Although it may seem less practical, it may be worth the trouble if you are participating in multiple training sessions per day or in multiple sports. For athletes who are just training once per day, a more realistic approach might be having your postworkout snack, and then following that with a balanced meal one to two hours later.

For effective postworkout fueling, consider what kind of snacks you could grab on your way out the door or even keep in your backpack or locker (if they're nonperishable). Snacks that have about 60 grams of carbohydrate include the following:

2 cups cereal + 1 cup milk

Yogurt + 1/2 cup granola + banana

1 Clif bar + 2 clementines

16 fl oz chocolate milk + apple

1 ready-to-drink protein shake (e.g., Gatorade, Muscle Milk, Core Power—varieties with 40 g CHO) + granola bar

Carbohydrate Loading

Considering that glycogen depletion particularly limits endurance performance, it should come as no surprise that endurance athletes are interested in delaying glycogen depletion as long as possible. Carbohydrate loading, sometimes referred to as *glycogen supercompensation*, can do just that, and has been shown to extend steady-state exercise by about 20 percent and improve endurance performance by 2 to 3 percent, though not all data supports similar findings. For instance, Burke et al. (2000) failed to find significant performance improvements in endurance cyclists when comparing carbohydrate loading and placebo groups. Carbohydrate loading enables an athlete to maintain high-intensity exercise for longer, but does not begin to affect the pace until after the first hour. These benefits are limited to well-trained endurance athletes; research has shown that carbohydrate loading does not benefit athletes competing in events lasting less than 90 minutes and could even negatively affect performance (Burke et al. 2002). There is also no research to show that carbohydrate loading can positively affect muscle size, despite some popularity in aesthetic sports like bodybuilding. More detail on carbohydrate loading will be discussed in chapter 10.

The Fad Diet Trap

"But when I don't eat carbohydrate, I lose weight!" As a dietitian I hear this kind of feedback all the time, and it's true. When you limit or don't eat carbohydrate at all, you *will* lose weight. However, the part that most people don't mention is that the weight loss is very much temporary. Let's break down what happens when you eat (or don't eat) carbs. When you consume carbohydrate your body digests it and breaks it down into simple sugars. As discussed earlier in this chapter, some of those simple sugars are stored as fuel. In order for your body to store that fuel, however, it must combine that simple sugar with water to form the molecule glycogen. This glycogen molecule of sugar and water quite literally weighs something. The average person who is eating adequate carbohydrate probably has 5 to 10 pounds (2-4.5 kg) of glycogen in their body, depending on body size.

When you limit carbohydrate, you pretty quickly burn through that stored glycogen, especially if you are very active—and therefore lose those first 5 to 10 pounds fairly quickly. It's for this reason that people who are limiting carbohydrate feel like their new diet worked and that carbs must be causing them to gain weight. For the same reason, they usually regain that 5 to 10 pounds pretty quickly once they regularly eat carbs again, further reinforcing that carbs are bad for them and that they shouldn't eat them. In reality, that 5- to 10-pound fluctuation is simply water weight.

The Keto Diet

The most extreme approach surrounding carbohydrate is the ever-popular ketogenic diet, often shortened to *keto*. The keto diet is a very low-carbohydrate, low-protein, high-fat diet that—if followed very strictly over many weeks—can cause the body to shift into ketosis. By definition, ketosis is a metabolic state that occurs when the body begins utilizing fat for energy instead of glucose. From an evolutionary standpoint, this function provides fuel for the body when food is scarce to help avoid starvation—but like so many things, humans have found a way to engineer this response deliberately. Because so many of the facts about the diet have become watered down as it has been sensationalized in the media, it's important to understand the mechanism of how keto does (and doesn't) work. The keto diet was originally developed as a treatment for epilepsy and is often effective in helping these patients. It has also been shown to be effective for treating certain types of brain tumors. Somewhere along the way, however, it was gobbled up by mainstream health and fitness media and has been touted as a weight-loss miracle, along with myriad other health claims.

As described previously, there is a clear reason that this diet causes initial weight loss: Glycogen depletion followed by a much smaller group of available foods tends to lead to a caloric deficit. Keto is also high in fat, which can be very satiating and decrease appetite. I like to bring athletes' attention to the high-fat aspect, which is often overlooked. Many people think they are following a ketogenic diet when they simply limit carbohydrate, but it is much more involved than that. A true ketogenic diet limits carbohydrate to very low amounts (usually recommended to be <50 g/day, sometimes as low as 10 g/day), is fairly low in protein (when carbohydrate is not present in adequate amounts the body uses a process called *gluconeogenesis* to convert protein into carbohydrate), and very high in fat. Hence, limiting carbohydrate to very low amounts but eating a lot of meat and other protein is not likely to induce ketosis. Additionally, to truly shift metabolism into ketosis, this very strict diet must be followed for up to four to six weeks, during which many people experience symptoms similar to the flu (commonly referred to as *keto flu*). Lastly, to truly be in ketosis requires complete adherence to the diet, with no wiggle room—a cheat meal will throw the body out of ketosis.

If ketosis is truly achieved and sustained, there is adequate research to support that it can lead to weight loss and in some cases improved blood glucose and other labs. However, there is very little research that sheds light on the long-term effects of following a ketogenic diet over decades. There is also no research to support that ketosis improves performance. There is some literature that has found endurance athletes in ketosis can perform as well as endurance athletes utilizing a high-carbohydrate diet, but there has yet to be research that shows superior performance. For example, Burke and colleagues (2017) found that the ketogenic diet impaired exercise economy of elite race walkers during intense training and negated the performance benefits that the athletes gained from intensified training.

Furthermore, if done poorly, the keto diet may actually decrease performance and health. First, the high-fat component can cause GI distress for some, which negatively affects performance and possibly interferes with adequate hydration. Second, the high saturated fat and cholesterol content of many keto-approved foods can actually lead to worsened lipid labs, which can ultimately harm cardiac health. With this in mind, and considering how difficult it is to achieve and sustain ketosis—especially with the busy schedule and travel that many athletes experience—I do not recommend that athletes follow a keto diet.

Another Day, Another Diet

Although the ketogenic diet is the most extreme approach to limiting carbohydrate, it is far from the only diet that does so. Paleo, the carnivore diet, and even Whole30, which all come with their own host of health-boosting claims, ultimately boil down to a similar weight-loss function: They all limit, to varying extents, foods and food groups that are rich in carbohydrate. The same could be said for some of the age-old diets like Atkins, South Beach, and the Dukan diet. All of these promote weight loss by limiting carbohydrate and overall calories.

In fact, though carbohydrate is often an easy target, the reality is that practically all fad diets are just different spins on the same end goal using different packaging and health claims. Eliminating various foods (and in some cases entire food groups) all leads to the same conclusion: a caloric deficit. Eating fewer calories than you were before you started the diet, over time, will lead to weight loss (especially if energy expenditure is higher than intake). Unfortunately, if a diet is not sustainable, the weight loss will not be either. Nearly 100 percent of diets fail long term, often with the dieter ultimately gaining back even more weight than they initially lost. This can lead to the diet cycling that so many get caught in, which causes frustration and can be detrimental to both physical and mental health. For these reasons, I recommend a diet that includes every food group—one that you can sustain over a lifetime, not just a few weeks, months, or even years.

Breaking Down Carbohydrate Misinformation

Finally, it's worth breaking down the myth that carbohydrate is "fattening." It's true that certain carbohydrate-rich foods have more fat than others. For instance, most desserts are high in both simple carbohydrate and fat. However, many carbohydrate-rich foods have gained a bad reputation that is not deserved, such as pasta, bread, and potatoes. The truth is that this carbohydrate breaks down to the same simple sugars as those in perceived "healthy" options like brown rice, quinoa, and sweet potatoes. As discussed thoroughly in this chapter, carbohydrate is necessary—often in much higher amounts than is commonly conveyed in the media.

That said, it's worth acknowledging a couple of ways in which carbohydrate can be sneaky. Although pasta, bread, and potatoes are inherently just as healthy as their counterparts, I challenge you to think about *how* you eat them. It's common to eat pasta with high-fat sauces like Alfredo or other cheese- or cream-based sauces and to top with additional cheese. We often spread bread with butter or dip it in oil and top potatoes with butter, cheese, bacon bits, and more. We also commonly pair carbohydrate-heavy foods with each other—for instance, a large plate of pasta and with garlic bread on the side or pizza with breadsticks. It's easy to see how additional calories and fat could quickly add up in these scenarios! Although it is important to get adequate carbohydrate, if you consistently combine or load up your carb-rich foods with high-fat sauces and toppings, it's easy to see how you could end up consuming excessive carbohydrate and ultimately calories. However, this is not unique to carbohydrate and would be true of any of the three macronutrients. Excess calories are excess calories, and any macronutrient that is chronically consumed in excess will be stored as fat.

Ultimately, athletes should not fear carbohydrate, but rather view it as a tool to help maximize performance. By considering your overall carbohydrate needs, properly timing intake before and after performance, and choosing the right types for the right situations, you can capitalize on all the energy-boosting benefits carbohydrate has to offer!

CHAPTER 4
Recover Faster With Protein

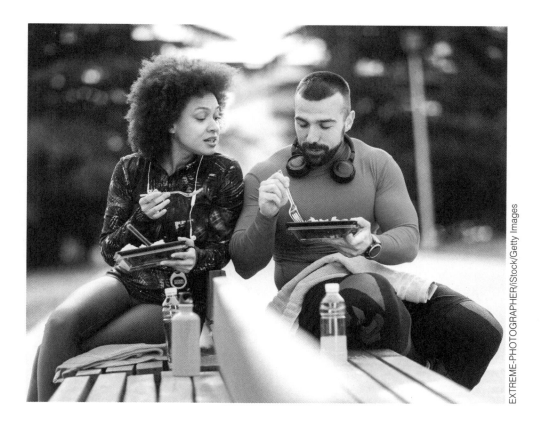

EXTREME-PHOTOGRAPHER/iStock/Getty Images

The second macronutrient, protein, is not only the primary building block for muscles and other cells, but also an integral piece of many antibodies and enzymes. Proteins are organic compounds made of amino acids. When you eat protein-rich food, your body breaks it down into individual amino acids, which can then be used as building blocks for muscles and other cells, as well as for many other important bodily functions (figure 4.1). Although it is often associated with the ability to build mass, particularly for athletes, protein helps promote good immune function and support a healthy metabolism. Protein also helps promote the feeling of fullness (called *satiety*) as a result of its slower digestion rate. Just like carbohydrate, 1 gram of protein yields 4 calories when digested.

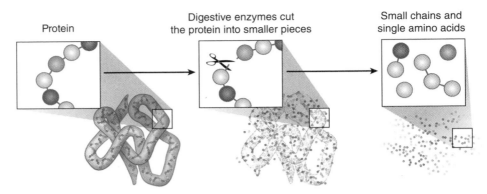

FIGURE 4.1   A protein molecule is digested and broken down into individual amino acids.

Reprinted by permission from G. Cardwell, *Gold Medal Nutrition*, 5th ed. (Champaign, IL: Human Kinetics, 2012), 6.

Recall from figure 3.1 that protein contributes very little to fueling any kind of exercise. Although muscle can be thought of as stored protein, you can avoid breaking down any additional muscle for fuel (sometimes referred to as *protein sparing*) with adequate carbohydrate on board. However, protein is a versatile macronutrient that can also be converted to glucose through a process called *gluconeogenesis* if carbohydrate intake is inadequate.

Types and Sources of Protein

Before diving into the practical application of protein on your plate, it's important to understand the differences in the types of protein. Although all proteins are made of individual amino acids, they are not all made of the same amino acids. Specifically, not all proteins contain essential amino acids, so named because they cannot be produced by the body and must come from diet. Foods with all nine essential amino acids (histidine, isoleucine, leucine, lysine, methionine, phenylalanine, threonine, tryptophan, and valine) are called *complete proteins*. Examples of complete proteins include animal products such as fish, beef, pork, poultry, eggs, and dairy, as well as some plant-based sources such as soy (tofu and edamame), quinoa, buckwheat, and hempseed, though these plant-based sources will not contain as much protein per serving as animal sources. Most plant-based sources of protein are considered incomplete proteins. This means they are completely lacking or are very low in one or multiple essential amino acids. With this in mind, you will need to be especially vigilant about getting enough of the right proteins if you exclude meat or animal products from your diet; this will be discussed in more depth later in the chapter.

Other Notable Amino Acids

All of the following amino acids are commonly found in supplemental form, but it's important to remember that if you are consuming adequate protein from varied sources, you are likely getting ample amino acids in your diet. When it comes to supplementation, more does not necessarily mean better (see recommendations made in chapter 8 for more detail).

- *Leucine.* One essential amino acid in particular gets a lot of attention when it comes to muscle protein synthesis, and deservedly so. A review by Norton and Layman (2006) concluded that leucine supplementation following exercise can enhance the stimulation of MPS, leading to greater muscle growth and repair. Many foods are high in leucine, notably animal products like meat, seafood, and dairy (not surprisingly, as these are high in amino acids in general), but another popular leucine-rich food is whey protein. Whey protein can be easily consumed in a shake or protein bar, making it a popular postworkout choice. Whey and other protein supplements will be discussed further in chapter 8.

- *Branched-chain amino acids (BCAAs).* In addition to leucine, the other two BCAAs, valine and isoleucine, have also been shown to improve endurance performance and reduce muscle damage.

- *Arginine.* Arginine is a precursor to nitric oxide, which helps dilate blood vessels and improve blood flow. This can enhance exercise performance by increasing oxygen and nutrient delivery to the muscles.

- *Glutamine.* Glutamine is important for muscle recovery and immune function, both of which can affect exercise performance. It has also been shown to increase muscle glycogen stores and improve hydration status.

- *Beta-alanine.* Beta-alanine is a precursor to carnosine, which helps buffer acid in the muscles during exercise and delay fatigue. It has been shown to improve high-intensity exercise performance.

Although meat is a great source of protein, it is far from the only one. Table 4.1 highlights foods that are rich in protein. The sources shown are fairly lean, meaning they have minimal amounts of fat compared to the amount of protein in a given serving size. There are also plenty of high-fat protein sources, such as bacon, sausage, salami, pepperoni, ribs, chicken with the skin on, high-fat cuts of beef, and fried meats. These foods can still be good sources of protein; however, because of their high fat content and for the purposes of nutrient timing, I recommend

TABLE 4.1   Lean, Protein-Rich Foods

Protein source	Portion size (oz)	Protein content (g)	Calories (kcal)	Cholesterol (mg)	Saturated fat (g)
Chicken breast, skinless, baked	3	26	128	73	0.6
Salmon, baked	3	22	206	63	1.2
Beef, top sirloin, broiled	3	23	207	78	4.8
Pork tenderloin, roasted	3	22	125	62	1.1
Tuna, canned in water	3	16	70	35	0.0
Greek yogurt, plain, nonfat	5.3	12	120	6	0.0
Cottage cheese, low fat	8	23	200	36	3.6
Lentils, boiled	4	9	115	0	0.0
Quinoa, cooked	8	8	156	0	0.6
Tempeh, cooked	8	31	320	0	3.7

limiting these options. Finding a balance of including these tasty higher-fat proteins from time to time while more often choosing leaner options is a good approach.

Protein Needs for Athletes

The total amount of protein you need per day depends on your body size as well as the type of activity you engage in. The protein you eat contributes to a positive protein balance, whereas training—especially resistance training—contributes to a negative protein balance. It's important to meet protein recommendations based on your activity level to help ensure that you end in a net positive protein balance. However, it's also important to remember that eating protein in excess of the recommended amounts, and in excess of what your body needs, does not translate to additional muscle mass.

Table 4.2 will help you calculate your protein needs based on activity. Although these recommendations are commonly accepted, it's important to note that some professionals recommend up to 2.0 grams per kilograms per day of protein for athletes engaging in resistance training. The recommendations do not vary by sex or gender.

Once you've estimated your total daily needs, take that number and divide it by the total number of meals and snacks that you generally eat in a day. This will give you an estimated number of grams of protein to aim for at each meal and snack. Remember, if you get stressed by spending

TABLE 4.2   Protein Recommendations Based on Type of Training

Type of training	Example of activity	Protein recommendation (g/kg)
Endurance (mostly aerobic based)	Running, swimming, cycling, rowing	1.2-1.4
Resistance (mostly strength based)	Sports that rely mostly on explosive movements such as jumping, sprinting, throwing, or hitting	1.6-1.7

Adapted by permission from E. Rosenbloom and J. Coleman, *Sports Nutrition: A Practice Manual for Professionals*, 5th ed., edited by C. Karpinski and C.A. Rosenbloom (Chicago: Academy of Nutrition and Dietetics, 2012).

too much time looking at specific numbers or counting calories or macronutrients, a good general goal can be to try to eat somewhere between 20 and 40 grams of protein at every meal and snack. Another common recommendation is to aim for 0.25 grams of protein per kilogram per meal. The following are a few examples of some foods that have between 20 and 40 grams of protein:

- 4 oz of chicken breast (32 g PRO)
- 2 cups of Cheerios with 2 cups of milk (22 g PRO)
- 3 oz tuna (24 g PRO)
- 2 cups of cooked beans (31 g PRO)
- 4 oz ground beef (28 g PRO)
- 1 scoop of 100 percent whey protein (~25 g PRO)

What About Injury?

It is generally agreed upon that recovering from injury requires additional protein—anywhere from 1.2 to 2.0 grams per kilogram per day, according to Beelen and colleagues (2010). The International Society of Sports Nutrition Position Stand on Protein and Exercise (Jager 2017) suggests a protein intake of 1.5 to 2.0 grams per kilogram per day for athletes with soft-tissue injuries to promote recovery and prevent muscle loss and 2.0 to 3.0 grams per kilogram per day for athletes with bone injuries to support bone healing and collagen synthesis. However, it's important to note that protein needs may vary depending on the individual athlete, the severity of the injury, and other factors such as age, training status, body weight, and level of physical activity. It's always best to consult with a sports dietitian for personalized recommendations when recovering from injury.

Protein Timing

Similarly to carbohydrate, consistently having protein present in your diet is incredibly important—arguably more important than the total amount of protein consumed. One of the most common missteps athletes make is focusing too heavily on postworkout protein or having most of their protein intake come from one meal (commonly dinner, which is more likely to include meat than other meals). Although the total amount of protein intake is important, it's vital to remember that MPS doesn't just happen after a lift or workout—it happens all day long. With this in

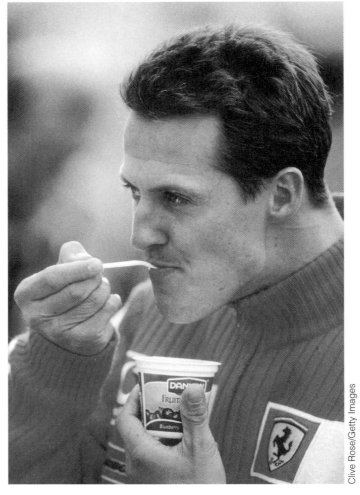

Clive Rose/Getty Images

Quick, on-the-go sources of protein like yogurt, beef jerky, and protein bars can be convenient for busy athletes.

mind, it's important to provide your body with the amino acids necessary to build and repair muscle mass by eating adequate amounts of protein throughout the day. An early study comparing subjects in a fasted and fed state found that MPS doubled in skeletal muscle among the fed subjects (Rennie et al. 1982).

Continued research on the subject has remained supportive of the notion that protein distribution across a day is important. A study by Mamerow et al. (2014) examining the effects of varied distributions of protein intake found that evenly distributing intake throughout the day increased MPS rates by 25 percent compared to a skewed distribution even though total intake was the same. Another study by Hudson and colleagues (2020) found that consuming a protein-rich meal every three hours throughout the day led to greater MPS compared to consuming the same amount of protein in fewer, larger meals.

Before the Workout

Although a preworkout meal should have a moderate amount of lean protein three to four hours from activity, the closer you get to competition, the more you should limit protein and focus on carbohydrate intake. The concept of including protein before a workout is a bit controversial: Some research has shown increased MPS when subjects ingested 20 grams of protein prior to a workout—specifically, high-quality protein that provides around 6 grams of essential amino acids (Tang et al. 2009). However, research by Tipton and colleagues (2007) showed that both preworkout and postworkout protein ingestion elicited similar MPS responses.

As the research stands right now, it likely depends on individual responsiveness to protein timing. Because of the propensity of protein to cause GI upset, if you are an hour or less away from activity, I would recommend limiting protein consumption to 15 grams or less and definitely avoid any high-fat proteins. This is especially true if your stomach is sensitive to eating prior to working out or if you are participating in high-intensity or endurance exercise. If you are participating in strength training, however, it may be helpful to include small amounts of protein in addition to carbohydrate in the hour leading up to your workout. A bigger athlete might also be able to tolerate more than the suggested 15 grams of protein, and some athletes may find certain high-protein foods don't bother their stomach at all and help keep them full for a long workout. As with many other things, recommendations may be subject to your individual tolerance. This is one of many reasons I suggest that you trial your fueling plan during training so that you learn what works well for you and what doesn't well ahead of competition.

During the Workout

It is not advised to consume protein during most workouts because of the slow digestion rate and the likelihood of GI upset. Additionally, research does not support that including protein during training or competition results in increased performance. As an exception, athletes participating in ultraendurance races or training for more than five hours per day should consume protein during this exercise in small quantities that will not cause GI upset. Although there is not research to support a performance benefit for doing so, this practice increases the protein available for recovery and MPS outside of training. More information on fueling ultraendurance races can be found in chapter 10.

After the Workout

As mentioned in chapter 3, both carbohydrate and protein are vitally important in the time that elapses after finishing a workout or competition. Biolo and colleagues (1997) were some of the first to conclude that protein intake immediately after exercise may be more anabolic than when ingested at some later time. In an analysis of 23 studies, Schoenfeld, Aragon, and Krieger (2013) concluded that consuming protein within a few hours of resistance exercise promotes MPS and enhances muscle growth and strength. Phillips and Van Loon (2011) also found that consuming protein during the postexercise recovery period can stimulate MPS and recommend consuming 20 to 25 grams of high-quality protein after exercise to optimize this response. However, interpreting the exact timing needs can be challenging due to the conflicting nature of the research. It is generally agreed that the efficiency of MPS diminishes as time elapses postworkout—one example from MacDougall and colleagues (1992) found that MPS was increased 2.5-fold at one hour after exercise and returned to baseline levels by six hours after exercise in untrained individuals. Protein supplementation within the first three hours of finishing exercise was also found to promote muscle recovery, gains in strength, and increases in muscle mass (Cribb and Hayes 2006). However, as pointed out by Areta and colleagues (2013), total daily protein intake distributed throughout the day is likely the most important factor in optimizing training adaptations.

From a practical standpoint, I encourage athletes to try to eat 20 to 40 grams of protein paired with carbohydrate within about an hour of finishing a workout. Although waiting longer won't negate the benefits of a postworkout snack, getting something in within that first hour will help you take advantage of the anabolic window created from the

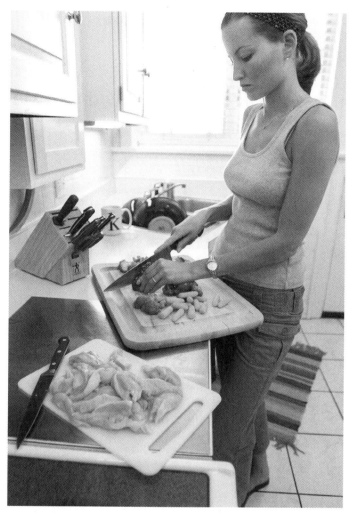

In addition to consuming protein in smaller amounts throughout the day, pairing a larger serving of protein alongside carbohydrate as part of a postworkout meal will maximize your anabolic window.

workout. This can also make it more likely that you get enough total calories to promote recovery, because most athletes will have a bigger meal one to three hours after finishing the workout and further capitalize on this window.

The importance of planning ahead for postworkout snacks is discussed in chapter 3, but it's worth reiterating here because protein can be even more challenging than carbohydrate to pack ahead or get on the go. Because many protein-rich foods like meat, seafood, and dairy are not shelf-stable and require refrigeration, your schedule, facilities, or travel logistics might make these options unrealistic. For this reason, convenience products like protein shakes and bars can be incredibly helpful for this time frame. For more specific postworkout recommendations, turn to chapter 9.

Vegan and Vegetarian Considerations

When specific food groups are excluded from your diet, particular attention should be given to making sure that you're getting adequate nutrients. For example, certain nutrients like protein, iron, B vitamins, calcium, zinc, and omega-3 fatty acids are found more abundantly and in more bioavailable forms in animal-based products and may not be consumed in adequate amounts if you limit or abstain from these products.

It's important to assess which nutrients you may be at risk of underconsuming if you decide to follow a restricted diet. The most restrictive diet is vegan, which includes no meat or animal-based products whatsoever, including dairy, eggs, and even honey, gelatin, and certain food dyes. Vegetarian refers to a slightly less restrictive approach that generally involves abstaining from meat and other animal products, though some vegetarians may still choose to consume eggs and milk. Pescatarian is the least restrictive of these approaches, allowing seafood but no other meat. Sometimes *plant-based* is used interchangeably with *vegan* or *vegetarian*, but technically this just refers to a diet that includes a lot of fruits, vegetables, grains, and legumes (similar to the Mediterranean diet) and does not necessarily mean abstaining from meat. Regardless of title, it's important to acknowledge the shortcomings in any limited diet and put purposeful effort toward getting nutrients through other foods—especially protein.

If you are only restricting meat then you should make an effort to include seafood, dairy, and eggs often. However, if you are restricting most or all of these groups of food you should be very conscious of including other protein-rich foods such as beans, legumes, lentils, edamame, soy milk, tofu, pea protein, quinoa, brown rice, and whole-wheat pasta, and even nuts, seeds and nut butters (which are not considered excellent sources of protein, but can help contribute toward your total). Eating a variety of plant-based protein sources will ensure that you are getting adequate amounts of all the essential amino acids. Some good plant-based sources of protein are shown in table 4.3.

Those who follow a vegetarian or vegan diet sometimes do so in an effort to eat a healthier diet overall. It's important to acknowledge that limiting meat and other animal products can improve some markers of health, including lowered intake of dietary fat, sodium, and other preservatives used in some meat products. However, it's also important to acknowledge that not everything about a meat-free diet is healthier. First, as just discussed, you can put yourself at risk of inadequate nutrient

TABLE 4.3   Protein Content of Vegetarian Protein Sources

Source	Amount (g per 100 g)
Vital wheat gluten	75.2
Seaweed (dried)	57.4
Hemp seeds	31.6
Peanuts	25.8
Almonds	21.1
Pistachio nuts	20.2
Tempeh	18.5
Pumpkin seeds	18.5
Flaxseed	18.3
Sesame seeds	17.7
Oats	16.9
Chia seeds	16.5
Cashews	15.3
Walnuts	15.2
Hazelnuts	14.9
Brazil nuts	14.3
Pine nuts	13.7
Soybeans	12.4
Buckwheat groats	11.7
Rye grain	10.3
Wheat flour	9.6
Lentils	9.0
Black beans	8.9
Chickpeas	8.9
Kidney beans	8.7
Tofu (firm)	8.2
Navy beans	8.2
Fava beans	7.6
Adzuki beans	7.5
Mung beans	7

Data from: VegFAQs; Available: https://vegfaqs.com/wp-content/uploads/2019/11/vegan-nutrition-chart-revised-1.png.

intake. Additionally, meat alternatives (for which options are increasing) are in many ways less healthy than their real-meat counterparts as a result of high amounts of sodium, sugar, and preservatives. For most people, good health and performance is most achievable and enjoyable by having a balanced diet that includes everything in moderation.

However, if you feel passionately about avoiding certain animal products for any reason, you should do so—just make sure you do so purposefully.

Much like carbohydrate, protein consumption is vitally important to your success as an athlete. Nutrient timing around protein can play an important role in maximizing muscle growth and recovery, and being purposeful with your protein choices can ensure you bounce back quicker from workouts and are ready to take on the next challenge. Protein also plays a role in supporting your immune system and preventing injury, which helps keep you on the field of play. Paying attention to this aspect of your diet is one of the best things you can do to continue to elevate your game.

CHAPTER 5
Meet Energy Needs With Fat

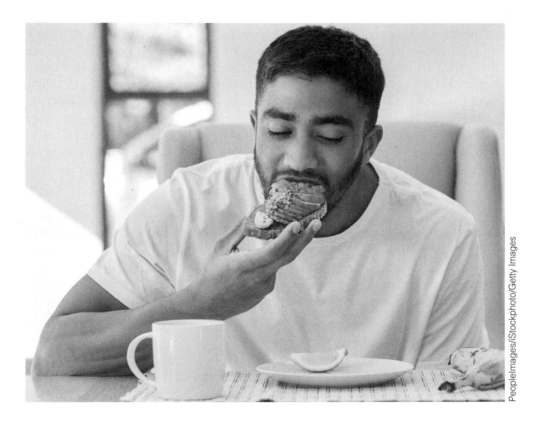

The third and final macronutrient to be discussed is fat. Many people naturally assume that fat is inherently bad because so much media attention has been given over the years to low-fat diets and criticism of body fat. However, fat plays a vital role in many bodily functions such as absorbing fat-soluble vitamins, synthesizing hormones, and being a source of essential fatty acids (fats that cannot be produced by the body and therefore must be obtained from diet). A certain amount of stored body fat is also a necessary structural component to protect vital organs and help keep you warm. Finally, fat is an important source of energy, and compared to the 4 calories per gram that carbohydrate and protein provide, 1 gram of fat rings in at 9 calories. Although fat can quickly add up to excess if consumed in high amounts and become stored as adipose tissue (commonly referred to as *body fat*), when used purpose-fully it can contribute to satiety and be helpful in keeping up with the caloric demands of being an athlete.

Types and Sources of Fat

As mentioned, fat tends to get a bad rap. This is partly because many high-fat foods are generally considered to be junk food. However, it's important to distinguish the difference between the different kinds of dietary fat, because some are bad for health, and some are actually very good for health. For example, cholesterol is a type of fat that is carried in the blood by molecules called *lipoproteins*. There are two main types of lipoproteins that carry cholesterol: low-density lipoprotein (LDL) and high-density lipoprotein (HDL). LDL cholesterol is often referred to as *bad cholesterol* because it can build up in the walls of arteries, leading to atherosclerosis (the hardening and narrowing of arteries). This can increase the risk of heart disease and stroke.

On the other hand, HDL cholesterol is often referred to as *good cholesterol* because it helps remove LDL cholesterol from the arteries and brings it back to the liver, where it can be broken down and removed from the body. Having higher levels of HDL cholesterol is associated with a lower risk of heart disease and stroke (AHA 2021a). The following sections will outline the different types and sources of these fats.

Trans Fat

Trans fat is well known for being the worst kind of dietary fat. Created by chemically altering liquid oils to make them solid and more shelf-stable (so they won't go bad as quickly), trans fat is found in some fried foods, baked goods, and margarines or other spreads. In chemistry, "trans" refers to the orientation of functional groups or atoms in a molecule, and means that the groups or atoms are on opposite sites of a double bond or ring structure. This chemical alteration causes trans fat to have a linear shape that tends to stack up tightly and therefore build up in arteries. This raises LDL (bad cholesterol) levels and lowers HDL (good cholesterol) levels, increasing the risk for diabetes, heart disease, and stroke (American Heart Association 2017).

Less than 1 percent of your total calories should come from trans fat. You can determine the amount of trans fat in a particular packaged food by looking at the Nutrition Facts panel (American Heart Association 2017). Trans fats are less common than they once were since they were banned by the FDA in 2018. However, this can be misleading because a product is considered to have 0 grams of trans fat if it contains less than 0.5 grams of trans fat per serving, so it's possible that small amounts might sneak in, especially if you eat many foods that contain these small amounts of trans fat (commercial baked goods, shortening, microwave popcorn, frozen pizzas, fried foods, and stick margarine).

Saturated Fat

Saturated fat is also generally considered to be an unhealthy fat, although a certain amount of saturated fat in the diet is necessary. Similar to trans fat, the chemical structure of saturated fat makes it more apt to cluster and therefore block arteries (though not to the same extent as trans fat). Foods that are high in saturated fat include beef, pork, lard, cream, butter, cheese, and some baked and fried foods. Notably, saturated fat is solid at room temperature, which makes it easy to differentiate from unsaturated fat. For instance, butter (saturated fat) is solid at room temperature, unlike olive oil (unsaturated fat). This is also seen when you cook ground beef or pork—you can drain off the fat while it's hot, but if you let that drained grease sit until it cools, it will solidify.

The American Heart Association (AHA 2021a, 2021b) recommends that 5 to 6 percent of your total calories come from saturated fat, or somewhere between 10 and 30 grams of saturated fat per day for most people. You can evaluate saturated fat on the Nutrition Facts panel of most products.

Unsaturated Fat

The last kind of fat is unsaturated fat. This is considered to be healthy fat and may be either monounsaturated or polyunsaturated. These fats can help lower LDL (bad) cholesterol levels and increase HDL (good) cholesterol levels. Unsaturated fats have been shown to actually have health benefits, and they are good for heart and brain health as well as fighting inflammation (Calder 2013), which athletes tend to have a lot of as a result of strenuous training loads. Figure 5.1 organizes the types of fats according to their benefits or hazards.

What Is Inflammation?

Inflammation is a natural immune response to infection, injury, or irritation in the body. It is a complex process that involves the release of various chemical mediators, such as cytokines and prostaglandins, by the immune cells in the affected area. Inflammation, at its root, is a good thing—it's a protective response that helps the body fight harmful stimuli. However, chronic inflammation can lead to tissue damage and contribute to the development of many chronic diseases.

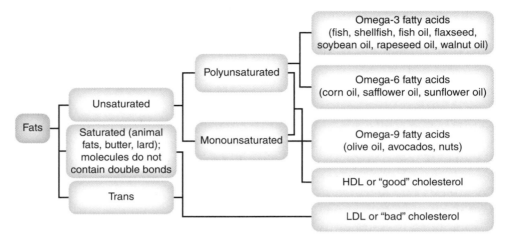

FIGURE 5.1   Types of good and bad fat.

Adapted from Murray and Kenney (2016).

Two types of polyunsaturated fats often garner the most attention: omega-3 and omega-6 fatty acids. These have similar benefits, but it can be helpful to still understand the distinction between them. Omega-3 and omega-6 fatty acids are both essential fatty acids, meaning that they must be obtained through diet. Omega-3 fatty acids are primarily found in fatty fish such as salmon, sardines, and mackerel, as well as in flaxseeds, chia seeds, and walnuts. Omega-6 fatty acids, on the other hand, are largely found in vegetable oils such as soybean oil, corn oil, and sunflower oil, as well as in nuts and seeds.

Some have inaccurately claimed that omega-6 fatty acids—specifically, seed oils—are inflammatory and bad for your health. In truth, it is recommended to maintain a balanced ratio of omega-6 to omega-3 fatty acids in the diet, because research suggests that consuming too much omega-6 relative to omega-3 is associated with increased inflammation and oxidative stress in healthy individuals (Simopoulos 2002). However, both omega-3 and omega-6 fatty acids are important for health. For example, a study by Mensink and colleagues (2003) found that replacing saturated fats with polyunsaturated fats, including seed oils such as sunflower and safflower oil, can reduce the risk of cardiovascular disease. This is a perfect example of how misinformation can create confusion and fear of perfectly safe foods.

Although these fats do have health benefits, they are still a fat and thus more calorically dense than the other macronutrients. For this reason, it's important to be purposeful when it comes to including fat in your diet and to try to include these healthy fats in moderation each day. The National Institutes of Health (2023) recommend that omega-6 fatty acids make up 0.6 percent of your total calories and omega-3 fatty acids 1.2 percent. It can be effective to supplement with a quality omega-3 supplement, especially depending on your access to foods rich in omega-3s. Supplements will be discussed in more detail in chapter 8.

Fat Needs for Athletes

As you'll recall from chapter 2, your balanced plate did not have a designated place for fat. This may seem surprising after having just discussed the necessity and health benefits of certain types of fats. However, fat tends to work itself into the diet through the other macronutrients, especially from proteins or a sauce or topping on a carbohydrate-rich food. Instead of designating a piece of your plate for fat, it is often a better approach to focus on including healthy fats daily. Table 5.1 lists

TABLE 5.1   Fats to Choose Often

Food	Serving size	Omega-3 fatty acid	Omega-6 fatty acid
NUTS AND SEEDS			
Almonds	28 g (1 oz)	0.001 g	3.36 g
Chia seeds	28 g (1 oz)	4.91 g	0.62 g
Flaxseeds	28 g (1 oz)	6.45 g	1.65 g
Hemp seeds	28 g (1 oz)	6.75 g	2.38 g
Pistachios	28 g (1 oz)	0.064 g	3.71 g
Walnuts	28 g (1 oz)	2.57 g	10.71 g
OILS			
Avocado oil	1 tbsp (14 g)	0.15 g	12.48 g
Canola oil	1 tbsp (14 g)	1.28 g	3.05 g
Coconut oil	1 tbsp (14 g)	0.008 g	0.07 g
Flaxseed oil	1 tbsp (14 g)	7.26 g	1.85 g
Olive oil	1 tbsp (14 g)	0.12 g	1.42 g
Safflower oil	1 tbsp (14 g)	0.13 g	10.09 g
Sunflower oil	1 tbsp (14 g)	0.93 g	9.88 g
SEAFOOD			
Herring	85 g (3 oz)	1.71 g	0.09 g
Salmon (farmed)	85 g (3 oz)	1.24 g	0.58 g
Salmon (wild)	85 g (3 oz)	1.52 g	0.41 g
Sardines	85 g (3 oz)	1.36 g	0.22 g
Trout	85 g (3 oz)	0.68 g	0.38 g

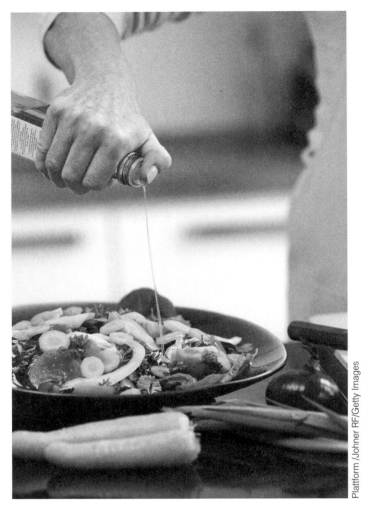

Plattform /Johner RF/Getty Images

Adding ingredients like olive oil to dishes can increase consumption of healthy omega-3 and omega-6 fatty acids.

some options for foods that are rich in omega-3 and omega-6 fatty acids. Table 5.2 lists some foods to limit or avoid; these are high in saturated or trans fat.

It's important to remember that when it comes to high-fat foods, limiting yourself does not mean you can *never* have them. In fact, completely restricting foods you enjoy often creates a strong psychological drive for them, leading you to either replace them with a similar food or eventually eat a large amount of the avoided food, sometimes even to the point of feeling like you're out of control. What tends to be a better approach is to include these foods as part of your regular routine.

TABLE 5.2   **Fats to Limit**

Food	Serving size	Saturated fat	Trans fat
Butter	1 tbsp	7.3 g	0.1 g
Margarine	1 tbsp	2.1 g	0.3 g
Lard	1 tbsp	5.0 g	0.5 g
Shortening	1 tbsp	3.2 g	1.7 g
Bacon	3 slices	4.5 g	0.3 g
Sausage	1 link	3.7 g	0.3 g
Beef (80% lean)	4 oz	7.3 g	0.3 g
Cheese	1 oz	5.5 g	0.1 g
Cream	1 tbsp	1.7 g	0.0 g
Whole milk	1 cup	4.6 g	0.0 g
Ice cream	1 cup	16.0 g	1.5 g
Cake	1 slice (1/12 of a 9-inch diameter)	5.3 g	0.2 g
Cookies	2 (2-inch diameter cookies	3 g	0.2 g
Frosted cake doughnut	1 doughnut	9 g	0.4 g
Fried chicken	1 breast	7 g	0.4 g
French fries	2 cups	4.0 g	0.5 g
Onion rings	10 pieces	6.0 g	0.5 g

Although this approach of including unhealthy but enjoyable foods applies to everyone, regardless of goals, it is fair to acknowledge that being purposeful with fat intake is helpful for reaching weight-related goals. Those with weight-loss goals still need to consume some fat—there are many bodily processes that rely on these baseline amounts of dietary fat—but because fat is calorie dense, choosing leaner options most of the time will help promote a calorie deficit. For those trying to gain weight, the caloric density of fat can help them achieve adequate intake without causing discomfort. However, this does not mean going crazy with all high-fat foods—it's still important to prioritize getting these additional calories from mostly healthy fats. You can find more information on both weight-loss and weight-gain strategies in chapter 12.

There are actually not specific recommendations for athletes when it comes to fat intake. Instead, it is recommended to use the acceptable macronutrient distribution range (AMDR) established by the Institute of Medicine (2002), which suggests that 20 to 35 percent of total calories come from fat; this is in line with what many athletes report consuming. From there more specific recommendations might be influenced

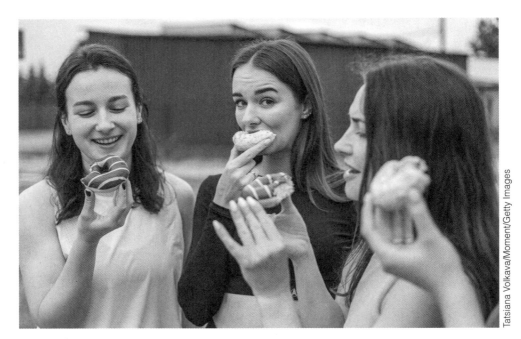

Tatsiana Volkava/Moment/Getty Images

While it is important to use moderation around foods that are high in unhealthy fats, they can still be part of a healthy balanced diet.

by training and body composition goals, although most can be accomplished within the AMDR. Although there certainly can be exceptions, long-term fat restriction can affect the ability to get adequate calories to support performance and health as well as the ability to absorb fat-soluble vitamins from the diet and obtain essential fatty acids. A review by Whittaker and Wu (2021) of 16 randomized controlled trials found that low-fat diets were associated with lower levels of testosterone and other important hormones in men. A study by Tomten and Hostmark (2006) also found fat intake among female endurance runners to be a major distinguishing factor between those athletes being healthy and having menstrual dysfunction. This study led to those authors making a recommendation that endurance athletes consume no less than 1 gram per kilogram per day of fat. If you are limiting fat to less than 20 percent of total calories, such restriction should be limited to short-term scenarios such as making weight for weight-class sports or limiting fat prior to competition due to GI concerns.

Some athletes may also seek out a very high-fat diet with the goal of metabolic adaptations that support burning fat for fuel instead of carbohydrate (generally summarized as a ketogenic diet). The keto diet was discussed in depth in chapter 3, but as a quick summary, to truly shift into ketosis metabolically requires a very high-fat, low-protein, low-carbohydrate diet that must be followed strictly with no lapse for many weeks. If ketosis is achieved, research has shown that athletes doing low- to moderate-intensity activity can perform as well as their counterparts eating a high-carbohydrate diet (Zajac et al. 2014). However, research has yet to show an improvement in performance. It has also been shown that such approaches limit an athlete's ability to excel at high-intensity exercise (Paoli et al. 2013). With this in mind, and because of the difficult nature of properly carrying out a ketogenic diet, I do not recommend this approach.

Fat Timing

When it comes to nutrient timing surrounding fat and performance, more research is still needed. Fat is slower to digest than its macro-nutrient counterparts, which isn't always helpful when it comes to athletic performance. Just like carbohydrate and protein, the exact amount of time that it takes fat to digest depends on many different factors, including the breakdown of fats and the composition of the rest of the meal. Generally speaking, fats that are high in unsaturated fatty acids tend to be digested more quickly than those that are high in saturated fatty acids.

The primary consideration at the present time is to try to limit fat in the hours leading up to training and competition and to keep fat intake during exercise as low as possible; this is especially true for athletes with sensitive stomachs. Because of its generally slow digestion rate, having too much fat before or during activity can lead to an upset stomach and uncomfortable GI symptoms that can hinder performance.

Diet Trends: Low Fat to Full Fat

Your body relies on fat the most during rest and light- to moderate-intensity exercise, and it also relies more on fat during endurance exercise once carbohydrate stores have been depleted (see figure 3.1 in chapter 3 for a good reference of this breakdown). In recent years research has focused on various approaches to leverage low-carbohydrate, high-fat diets with the goal of making the body more efficient at using fat. This strategy of training with low carbohydrate availability is usually referred to as *training low*. Although similar to the ketogenic diet discussed in chapter 3, this approach does not cause a true metabolic shift like keto does. An athlete who is training low would likely train in a fasted state, most commonly accomplished by exercising in the morning before they have had breakfast. Alternatively, they might attempt to deplete their glycogen stores in a morning training session before a second exercise session in the afternoon with the hope that their body would be more likely to rely on fat oxidation as opposed to carbohydrate, then have a glycogen-repleting meal after the second training session. It is widely agreed that a high-fat diet does cause a higher fat oxidation (i.e., burning) rate, but the impact on performance is less clear and should be studied further. A study by Impey and colleagues (2016) found that cyclists who trained with low muscle glycogen levels had improved time trial performance compared to those who trained with high muscle glycogen levels. However, there are also many studies that found no improvement in performance with this method as compared to a high-carbohydrate diet (Wynne et al. 2021).

Many researchers have sought to find a balance between the approaches and explored strategically using a high-fat diet. For example, Yeo and colleagues (2011) proposed consuming a diet of 70 percent fat and 15 percent carbohydrate for 5 to 14 days before an event, then using a traditional carbohydrate-loading approach right before competition, which would in theory increase fat oxidation rates but replenish glycogen stores. Ultimately, though, results were similar and performance enhancements were not significant. Similarly, Volek and colleagues (2016) found that 20 weeks of ahigh-fat diet improved fat oxidation considerably in ultraendurance runners, but glycogen utilization and repletion were similar to the high carbohydrate group during a 3-hour run.

Although there remains to be any research showing significant improvements in performance, there have been some studies that find small improvements. Among endurance athletes, Rowlands and Hopkins (2002) showed that an 11.5-day high-fat diet followed by a 2.5-day carbohydrate-loading regimen reported a nonsignificant 3 to 4 percent improvement during a 100-kilometer time trial. This study also found that the power output during the last 5 kilometers of this time trial was 1.3 times greater after the high-fat diet compared with the high-carbohydrate diet.

Overall, given how difficult it is to carry out a very specific diet like the ones just described, and how mixed the results in performance improvements (especially significant ones), I would not generally recommend this approach for most athletes. However, if you are competing in an endurance sport at a very high level, and you have the time, means, and support to carry out a very regimented diet like those described above, an approach like these might be worth looking into further.

Although fat receives significantly less attention than carbohydrate and protein when it comes to athletic performance, fat does play an important role in an athlete's diet. Fat is an essential macronutrient that provides a rich source of energy to support the high expenditure of an athlete. It plays an important role in regulating hormone levels, maintaining healthy immune function, and supporting the absorption of fat-soluble vitamins. Athletes should not fear fat, but rather look for ways to include healthy fats in their diet and be cognizant that they are not overdoing it on foods that are high in trans and saturated fat, which can negatively affect health if consumed in excess. Consideration should be given to the timing of those fats given their potential to cause GI distress during activity.

Now that you've learned about each of the three macronutrients and how they fit into a balanced diet, it's time to dial in a little bit further and discuss the role of micronutrients in promoting optimal performance for athletes.

CHAPTER 6
Elevate Performance With Vitamins and Minerals

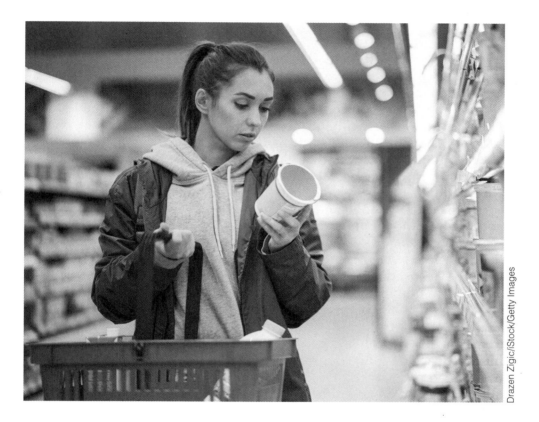

Drazen Zigic/iStock/Getty Images

Now that you have learned about the three macronutrients, let's turn now to micronutrients. Micronutrients are chemical elements or substances required in trace amounts for normal growth and development—more strictly speaking, micronutrients refer to vitamins and minerals. The processes that vitamins and minerals are involved in are vast and include energy metabolism, immune function, bone health, ocular health, blood clotting, muscle and nerve function, fluid balance, and oxygen transport—practically every bodily process is affected by vitamins and minerals in some way. Vitamins and minerals can generally be obtained in adequate amounts through diet. However, it is worth noting that some research shows that athletes have higher micronutrient needs than nonathletes, depending on the intensity, duration, and mode of exercise. Because many athletes have a limited diet as a result of preferences, allergies, budget, schedule, and time (to name a few), it is important to ensure adequate vitamin and mineral intake to promote optimal health and performance. Although vitamins are essential to health, however, they can be detrimental in excess. This chapter will discuss the functions of vitamins and minerals and recommendations for their intake.

Vitamins and Minerals in Food

A common misconception about vitamins and minerals is that they are bad for you or not utilized well by the body if taken in synthetic form. This is not the case. Synthetic forms of vitamins and minerals are chemically and structurally the same as naturally occurring ones in food. It is worth noting, however, that vitamins and minerals found in food do tend to be more bioavailable (which refers to the ability and rate at which a nutrient or substance can be absorbed) as a result of the chemical forms found in food and the synergistic effect of the micronutrients and other components of the food (fluid, fiber, and other macro- and micronutrients). For example, vitamin C helps the body absorb iron, so having a salad with vitamin C–rich veggies along with your steak can increase absorption of the iron in the meat. Similarly, fat is needed to absorb fat-soluble vitamins, so having that oil-based dressing on top of your salad actually helps your body absorb all the vitamin A, E, and K found in those veggies!

Although it's not always possible to get all the micronutrients you need from food, evaluating your diet should be the first line of action before jumping to supplementation. To give yourself the best chance of getting adequate vitamins and minerals in your diet, consider the following:

1. You must eat enough food overall. Inadequate caloric intake will make it nearly impossible to get all the micronutrients you need.

2. You need balanced plates that consistently have carbohydrates, protein, and fruits and vegetables—not to mention healthy fats. Each of these categories brings a different subset of vitamins and minerals to the table. Carbohydrate-rich foods tend to be high in B vitamins like thiamin, riboflavin, niacin, and folate as well as minerals like iron, magnesium, and selenium. Protein-rich foods tend to be high in iron, zinc, B vitamins, vitamin E, calcium, and phosphorus. Fruits and vegetables have a wide variety of vitamins and minerals, especially vitamins A, C, E, and K, not to mention a plethora of antioxidants (compounds that help protect the body's cells from harmful molecules called *free radicals*).

3. You should eat a variety of foods within each group. Although the groups have generally similar benefits, eating a variety of different carbohydrates, proteins, and fruits and veggies will ensure that you get a wide variety of nutrients. As an example, meat and seafood are rich in iron, B vitamins, and zinc; dairy products are rich in calcium, vitamin D, and phosphorus; and seafood is rich in fatty acids, iodine, and magnesium. All of these foods have protein, but each subset brings a unique group of micronutrients and subsequent benefits. Interestingly enough, similar-colored fruits and vegetables (e.g., a tomato and a strawberry) tend to have similar subsets of vitamins and minerals. With this in mind, you can probably imagine how getting a variety of colors in your diet can help promote getting a variety of vitamins and minerals.

Vitamins and Minerals From Supplements

Although it is possible to get adequate vitamins and minerals from diet—and you should strive to do so—there are a number of reasons this may not be possible. If you have a limited diet for any reason (whether because of a difficult schedule, religious or ethical beliefs, food allergies

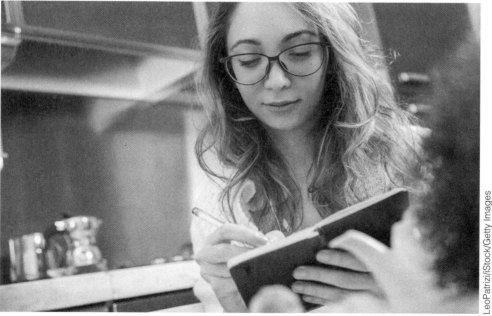

LeoPatrizi/iStock/Getty Images

Avoid taking individual nutrients in supplement form unless prescribed by a doctor or dietitian because of a documented deficiency or your diet has been evaluated and determined to be inadequate for a certain nutrient.

or intolerances, or you're just a picky eater) you should consider using a multivitamin supplement to help fill in any nutritional gaps.

If you do use a multivitamin supplement, it should be one that has undergone third-party testing through an agency such as USP, NSF, or Informed Sport (the importance of third-party testing for supplements will be discussed in much more detail in chapter 8). Using the proper multivitamin is a good way to help ensure that you are getting all the micronutrients your body needs without getting too much of any one micronutrient—because yes, you can get too much of a good thing! In fact, there are a number of vitamins and minerals that are dangerous to your health in very high doses. Reaching these levels would be nearly impossible to do through diet, but relatively easy to do if you're taking a supplement. Ultra-high doses are common in the supplement world, especially when using multiple supplements at once, and the body cannot regulate these high doses as easily in supplemental form. Because of this, I would not suggest taking an individual nutritional supplement unless prescribed by a doctor because of a documented deficiency or because your diet has been evaluated by a dietitian and determined to be inadequate for a certain nutrient.

Table 6.1 will briefly describe the different dietary reference intake definitions that will be used throughout this chapter. Recommendations will be given for each vitamin and mineral, as well as what each micronutrient is helpful for, what foods are rich in them, and general considerations to keep in mind for each.

TABLE 6.1 Dietary Reference Intake Definitions

Recommended dietary allowance (RDA)	Average daily level of intake sufficient to meet the nutrient requirements of nearly all (97%-98%) healthy individuals; often used to plan nutritionally adequate diets.
Adequate intake (AI)	Intake that is assumed to ensure nutritional adequacy; established when evidence is insufficient to develop an RDA.
Tolerable upper intake level (UL)	Maximum daily intake that is unlikely to cause adverse health effects. It is nearly impossible to reach the UL of any given nutrient from food; however, it is not uncommon for supplements to provide more than the UL, especially when multiple supplements are used.

Reprinted by permission from D. Benardot, *Advanced Sports Nutrition*, 3rd ed. (Champaign, IL: Human Kinetics, 2021).

These recommendations vary slightly based on age. Children, adolescents, and adults over age 65 should reference the guidelines specific to those age groups. Additionally, those who are pregnant or lactating should always reference values for these situations specifically.

Vitamins

There are two classes of vitamins: water soluble and fat soluble. Understanding the difference can be helpful when considering what vitamins might or might not be helpful to include as part of your routine. The class of vitamin also determines how much can be safely taken—a consideration often overlooked by a supplement-hungry public.

Water-Soluble Vitamins

The water-soluble vitamins are vitamin C and the B vitamins. *Water soluble* means that these vitamins bind to water within the body and therefore are excreted via urine. For that reason, it's harder to get "too much" of these vitamins because the body cannot use or store excess amounts and instead will just excrete them. Mega-doses of these water-soluble vitamins are incredibly common—I like to call them "expensive pee," because most of that mega-dose just ends up getting flushed down the toilet. However, it is still possible to get too much of these nutrients, and there can still be symptoms associated with doing so. For example, mega-doses of vitamin C can cause diarrhea and kidney stones.

Vitamin C

Vitamin C is a commonly discussed and supplemented water-soluble vitamin. Vitamin C is important for immune health and collagen synthesis and is an important antioxidant. Although many mammals can produce vitamin C, humans must obtain vitamin C from foods and other sources. It's contained in high concentration in fresh fruits and vegetables, especially citrus fruits. Vitamin C is one of the most widely used supplements and is commonly found in those mega-doses mentioned above. Because it's water soluble and can be cleared by the body, there is a low risk of health consequences from these high amounts, but it's important to note that *more* does not mean *better*. Getting an adequate amount of vitamin C is important for health, but getting extra does not provide additional health benefits and, as previously mentioned, can potentially cause health detriments.

It's incredibly common for people to start supplementing with vitamin C when they feel a cold coming on, but once you start experiencing symptoms, it is too late to receive the immune-supporting benefits of vitamin C. A better approach is to consistently include fruits and veggies rich in vitamin C—and if you can not, then supplement consistently, not just when you start to feel sick. Most multivitamins provide 100 percent of the recommended dietary allowance of vitamin C, which would be adequate for most people.

Vitamin C Timing

Many vitamins and minerals do not have a specific timing component, and is generally advised for athletes to take them at a time that works with their schedule and that they'll actually remember. For vitamin C, however, there is a school of thought that higher doses of vitamin C taken before a workout may actually blunt the training response, though there is limited research to support this. One study by Paulsen and colleagues (2014) found that high-dose vitamin C supplementation (1,000 mg/day) in combination with endurance training blunted certain cellular signaling pathways related to the body's ability to adapt to endurance exercise.

However, it's important to note that this study used a very high dose of vitamin C, and the findings may not necessarily apply to the moderate or lower doses typically found in standard vitamin C supplements or a balanced diet. More research is needed to fully understand the potential impact of vitamin C supplementation and timing on training adaptations.

From an athletic performance standpoint, vitamin C protects against oxidative stress, which is commonly associated with endurance and ultraendurance training. Although many studies have been conducted on the impact of vitamin C on performance and recovery, currently the research is conflicting and far from conclusive. With this in mind, an athlete's approach should be to meet the RDA and try to get plenty of vitamin C via their diet. Table 6.2 highlights the RDA and UL for vitamin C as well as foods rich in the nutrient.

TABLE 6.2   Vitamin C: Intake Guidelines and Food Sources

RDA	Males ages 19 and up: 90 mg
	Females ages 19 and up: 75 mg
UL	2,000 mg; taking more than this amount may cause GI distress and diarrhea
Foods rich in vitamin C	Citrus fruits (oranges, grapefruits, lemons), kiwi, bell peppers, Brussels sprouts, strawberries, tomatoes, broccoli, cauliflower, cabbage, white potatoes

Data from: National Institutes of Health Office of Dietary Supplments; Available: https://ods.od.nih.gov/Health-Information/nutrientrecommendations.aspx. Data from: Harvard T.H. Chan School of Public Health; Available: https://www.hsph.harvard.edu/nutritionsource/.

Vitamin B₁ (Thiamin)

Vitamin B$_1$, also called *thiamin*, plays a crucial role in the growth and function of various cells and is involved in many energy-producing reactions. Only small amounts are stored in the liver, so a daily intake of thiamin-rich foods is needed. It is not commonly supplemented unless as part of a B-vitamin complex. Research is fairly limited regarding thiamin and exercise, but some research suggests that higher amounts of thiamin may be needed when exercise intensity and duration increase. However, until the research is more conclusive, athletes should not aim to consume more than the RDA. Table 6.3 highlights the RDA and UL for thiamin as well as foods rich in the nutrient.

Vitamin B₂ (Riboflavin)

Vitamin B$_2$, known as *riboflavin*, is involved in many energy-producing reactions as well as the breakdown of fats, steroids, and medications. Bacteria in the gut can produce small amounts of riboflavin, but not enough to meet dietary needs. Similarly to thiamin, more research is

B Vitamin Supplements: Are They Worth the Hype?

B vitamins function as coenzymes, which means they play a crucial role in supporting various metabolic reactions in the body by working alongside important enzymes that convert food into energy. The B vitamins will be discussed individually, but with the exception of vitamin B$_6$ and vitamin B$_{12}$ they are not often supplemented individually. More often they are supplemented collectively as a B-complex vitamin.

B vitamins are incredibly common in the supplement world in oral form and increasingly in injectable form, and it's not uncommon to see doses that are thousands (sometimes even tens of thousands) in excess of the RDA for that vitamin. Because B vitamins are water soluble and excess amounts will simply be excreted in your urine, the risk of adverse effects from these mega-doses is low and these tend to only be a waste of money. However, even with water-soluble vitamins there is always some amount of risk with super high doses, and athletes might see side effects like headaches, diarrhea, and even kidney stones in extreme doses of Vitamin C.

As you learn about each B vitamin, you'll begin to see a trend that most of them are not needed in any dose that exceeds the normal recommendation. There are some situations that warrant supplementation of certain B vitamins, but as with any supplement you should choose a brand and product that is third-party tested (see chapter 8 for more information on this process).

TABLE 6.3   **Vitamin B₁ (Thiamin): Intake Guidelines and Food Sources**

RDA	Males ages 19 and up: 1.2 mg Females ages 19 and up: 1.1 mg
UL	None
Foods rich in vitamin B₁	Fortified breakfast cereals, pork, fish, beans, lentils, green peas, breads, noodles, rice, sunflower seeds, yogurt

Data from: National Institutes of Health Office of Dietary Supplments; Available: https://ods.od.nih.gov/Health-Information/nutrientrecommendations.aspx. Data from: Harvard T.H. Chan School of Public Health; Available: https://www.hsph.harvard.edu/nutritionsource/.

needed to definitively speak to the effects that exercise has on riboflavin in the body, but a study by Sato and colleagues (2011) reported no significant change in blood riboflavin concentrations in male and female participants when comparing off-season and intense in-season training. This would imply that riboflavin is not affected by exercise and that athletes should not require more than the RDA. Table 6.4 highlights the RDA and UL for riboflavin as well as foods rich in the nutrient.

TABLE 6.4   **Vitamin B₂ (Riboflavin): Intake Guidelines and Food Sources**

RDA	Males ages 19 and up: 1.3 mg Females ages 19 and up: 1.1 mg
UL	None
Foods rich in vitamin B₂	Milk, yogurt, cheese, eggs, lean beef and pork, organ meats (e.g., liver), chicken breast, salmon, fortified cereal and bread, almonds, spinach

Data from: National Institutes of Health Office of Dietary Supplments; Available: https://ods.od.nih.gov/Health-Information/nutrientrecommendations.aspx. Data from: Harvard T.H. Chan School of Public Health; Available: https://www.hsph.harvard.edu/nutritionsource/.

Vitamin B₃ (Niacin)

Vitamin B₃, also known as *niacin*, has over 400 enzymatic reactions that depend on it. Niacin helps convert nutrients into energy, create cholesterol and fats, and form and repair DNA, and it also has some antioxidant effects. The two most common forms of niacin in food and supplements are nicotinic acid and nicotinamide. The body can also convert tryptophan, an amino acid, to nicotinamide. A niacin deficiency is rare because it is found in many foods, both animal and plant based.

There is currently no research suggesting that higher amounts of niacin are needed for athletes. Despite this, it is not uncommon for supplements to include high doses of niacin, which can cause flushing and reddening of the face as well as itching. Table 6.5 highlights the RDA and UL for niacin as well as foods rich in the nutrient.

TABLE 6.5   Vitamin B₃ (Niacin): Intake Guidelines and Food Sources

RDA*	Males ages 19 and up: 16 mg NE Females ages 19 and up: 14 mg NE
UL	35 mg for all adults ages 19 and up
Foods rich in vitamin B₃	Beef, pork, poultry, fish, brown rice, fortified cereals and breads, nuts, seeds, legumes, bananas

*Niacin is measured in milligrams (mg) of niacin equivalents (NE). One NE equals 1 mg of niacin or 60 mg of tryptophan.

Data from: National Institutes of Health Office of Dietary Supplments; Available: https://ods.od.nih.gov/Health-Information/nutrientrecommendations.aspx. Data from: Harvard T.H. Chan School of Public Health; Available: https://www.hsph.harvard.edu/nutritionsource/.

Vitamin B₅ (Pantothenic Acid)

Vitamin B₅, or pantothenic acid, is used to make coenzyme A (CoA), a chemical compound that is vital for creating and breaking down fatty acids as well as other important metabolic functions. Bacteria in the gut can produce some pantothenic acid but not enough to meet dietary needs. Pantothenic acid is found in almost all plant and animal foods to some degree, because the vitamin is found in all living cells.

Some recent research has suggested that exercise may increase pantothenic acid needs, but the results have not been confirmed in human models. Athletes should aim to get the RDA for pantothenic acid. Table 6.6 highlights the RDA and UL for pantothenic acid as well as foods rich in the nutrient.

TABLE 6.6   Vitamin B₅ (Pantothenic Acid): Intake Guidelines and Food Sources

RDA	Males and females ages 19 and up: 5 mg
UL	None
Foods rich in vitamin B₅	Fortified cereals, organ meats (liver, kidney), beef, chicken breast, mushrooms, avocados, nuts, seeds, dairy milk, yogurt, potatoes, eggs, brown rice, oats, broccoli

Data from: National Institutes of Health Office of Dietary Supplments; Available: https://ods.od.nih.gov/Health-Information/nutrientrecommendations.aspx. Data from: Harvard T.H. Chan School of Public Health; Available: https://www.hsph.harvard.edu/nutritionsource/.

Vitamin B₆ (Pyridoxine)

Vitamin B₆, also called *pyridoxine*, has three major forms. Pyridoxal phosphate (PLP) is the active coenzyme form and most common measure of B₆ blood levels in the body. PLP assists over 100 different enzymes that have important functions such as breaking down proteins, carbohydrates, and fats; buffering other nutrients; and supporting immune function and brain health.

Like so many examples so far, research is conflicting as to whether vitamin B_6 needs are higher among athletes. However, Manore (2000) reports that inadequate vitamin B_6 intake can interfere with ability to perform optimally, and specifically that deficiency of vitamin B_6 negatively affects aerobic capacity. With this in mind, an athlete might want to ensure that B_6 levels are adequate if they are concerned about intake. Athletes who are vegetarian or vegan may be at greater risk for B_6 deficiency given that many foods rich in B_6 are animal products.

Vitamin B_6 is one of the more commonly individually supplemented B vitamins. Although there are some instances where a physician might prescribe a higher dose, caution should be used when supplementing vitamin B_6 due to the risk of toxicity. Table 6.7 highlights the RDA and UL for B_6 as well as foods rich in the nutrient.

TABLE 6.7   Vitamin B_6 (Pyridoxine): Intake Guidelines and Food Sources

RDA	Males ages 14-50: 1.3 mg Males ages 51 and up: 1.7 mg Females ages 14-18: 1.2 mg Females ages 19-50: 1.3 mg Females ages 51 and up: 1.5 mg
UL	100 mg for adults ages 19 and older, with slightly lesser amounts in children and teenagers
Foods rich in vitamin B_6	Beef liver, tuna, salmon, fortified cereals, chickpeas, poultry, dark leafy green vegetables, bananas, papayas, oranges, and cantaloupe

Data from: National Institutes of Health Office of Dietary Supplments; Available: https://ods.od.nih.gov/Health-Information/nutrientrecommendations.aspx. Data from: Harvard T.H. Chan School of Public Health; Available: https://www.hsph.harvard.edu/nutritionsource/.

Vitamin B_7 (Biotin)

Vitamin B_6, also called *biotin*, is commonly touted for its benefits to boost hair, skin, and nail health, though research showing a benefit of biotin supplementation is lacking. Like many B vitamins, it is involved in many important enzymatic reactions, including the breakdown of macronutrients. It also helps regulate genes and cell signaling.

Biotin is rarely mentioned in tandem with improved athletic performance, and there is no solid research to support that athletes need more biotin than nonathletes. Table 6.8 highlights the RDA and UL for B_7 as well as foods rich in the nutrient.

Vitamin B_9 (Folate)

Vitamin B_9, also called *folate*, is often added to foods and sold as a supplement in the form of folic acid, which is actually more bioavailable than folate in food sources. Folate plays a crucial role in growth and

TABLE 6.8   Vitamin B₇ (Biotin): Intake Guidelines and Food Sources

RDA	Males ages 19 and up: 30 mcg
	Females ages 19 and up: 30 mcg
UL	None
Foods rich in vitamin B₇	Beef liver, eggs (cooked), salmon, avocados, pork, sweet potato, nuts and seeds

Data from: National Institutes of Health Office of Dietary Supplments; Available: https://ods.od.nih.gov/HealthInformation/nutrientrecommendations.aspx. Data from: Harvard T.H. Chan School of Public Health; Available: https://www.hsph.harvard.edu/nutritionsource/.

development, specifically in forming DNA and RNA and in producing red blood cells that supply oxygen during times of rapid growth and development. For these reasons folate is usually most closely associated with its higher requirements for pregnant women. It is also vital in breaking down the amino acid homocysteine, which can be harmful in high amounts.

Folate is rarely mentioned in tandem with improved athletic performance, and there is no solid research to support that athletes need more folate than nonathletes. Table 6.9 highlights the RDA and UL for B₉ as well as foods rich in the nutrient.

TABLE 6.9   Vitamin B₉ (Folate): Intake Guidelines and Food Sources

RDA	Males ages 19 and up: 400 mcg DFE (dietary folate equivalents)
	Females ages 19 and up: 400 mcg DFE (dietary folate equivalents)
UL	1000 mcg/day
Foods rich in vitamin B₉	Dark leafy greens, beans, peanuts, sunflower seeds, fresh fruits, whole grains, liver, fish, seafood, eggs, fortified foods and supplements

Data from: Harvard T.H. Chan School of Public Health; Available: https://www.hsph.harvard.edu/nutritionsource/folic-acid/.

Vitamin B₁₂ (Cobalamin)

Vitamin B₁₂, sometimes called *cobalamin*, binds to protein and is essential to form red blood cells and DNA. It is also important in the function and development of brain and nerve cells. In the stomach, hydrochloric acid and enzymes unbind vitamin B₁₂ into its free form. From there, vitamin B₁₂ combines with a protein called *intrinsic factor* so that it can be absorbed further down in the small intestine.

Supplements and fortified foods contain B₁₂ in its free form so it may be more easily absorbed. A variety of vitamin B₁₂ supplements are available, including pills, powder, liquids, and sublingual forms. Although some claim that certain delivery methods are better for absorption, at this point studies have not shown a significant difference. Vitamin B_{12} tablets are available in dosages far exceeding the recommended dietary allowance, but absorption will be limited because an adequate amount of intrinsic factor is also needed.

Current research suggests that B_{12} supplementation is only needed if levels are deficient, though supplementation to correct a deficiency may improve athletic performance. Similarly to vitamin B_6, most dietary sources of vitamin B_{12} are of animal origin, so vegetarian and vegan athletes will likely benefit from supplementation. In cases of severe vitamin B_{12} deficiency as a result of inadequate intrinsic factor (pernicious anemia), doctors may prescribe intramuscular B_{12} injections.

Vitamin B_{12} and folate are very much interrelated in terms of their synthesis and metabolism. Because of this, high folate intake can mask B_{12} deficiency. Table 6.10 highlights the RDA and UL for B_{12} as well as foods rich in the nutrient.

TABLE 6.10   Vitamin B_{12} (Cobalamin): Intake Guidelines and Food Sources

RDA	Males and females ages 14 and up: 2.4 mcg
UL	None; however, some evidence suggests that supplements of 25 mcg or higher may increase the risk of bone fractures
Foods rich in vitamin B_{12}	Fish, shellfish, liver, red meat, eggs, poultry, dairy products (such as milk, cheese, and yogurt), fortified nutritional yeast, fortified breakfast cereals, enriched soy or rice milk

Data from: Harvard T.H. Chan School of Public Health; Available: https://www.hsph.harvard.edu/nutritionsource /vitamin-b12/.

Fat-Soluble Vitamins

Unlike water-soluble vitamins, fat-soluble vitamins are absorbed via fat in the diet and can be stored in the body. It's crucial to understand that you can absolutely get too much of these nutrients and most have serious consequences associated with doing so.

Vitamin A

Although vitamin A is most often associated with eye health, this vitamin is an important component of many other reactions in the body. Vitamin A helps build bone, regulate cell growth, stimulate white blood cells, and maintain healthy endothelial cells (cells that line the inner surface of blood vessels).

There are two main forms of vitamin A in the human diet: The first is preformed vitamin A (retinol and retinyl esters), which comes from animal products, fortified foods, and vitamin supplements. The other

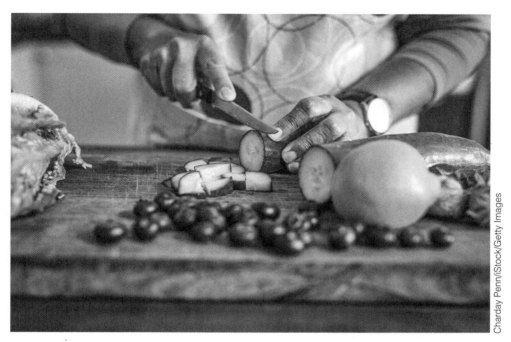

Charday Penn/iStock/Getty Images

Fruits and vegetables are a key source of vitamins and minerals in the diet.

form is provitamin A carotenoids that are converted to retinol, which are found naturally in plant foods, especially those that are orange, yellow, and red. Evidence suggests that eating a variety of foods rich in vitamin A, especially fruits and vegetables, has a protective effect against certain cancers and some diseases of the eye, though the health benefit of vitamin A supplements is less clear.

Many studies have been done on antioxidants and athletic performance and recovery. One study of competitive rowers by Braakhuis, Hopkins, and Lowe (2013) found that dietary intake of vitamin A was positively correlated to total antioxidant capacity, meaning that dietary vitamin A intake can have a positive impact on an athlete's ability to fight inflammation; however, they note that the exercise training itself was a more influential factor. Overall, more research is needed to pinpoint the specific effect of vitamin A. With this in mind, athletes should aim to consume the RDA, but should take special note to not exceed the UL to avoid toxicity. Although most supplements won't contain toxic levels of vitamin A on their own, it's not uncommon to get excess amounts when taking multiple supplements. Always ensure that you have accounted for the collective amounts of individual nutrients you're taking.

Historically, vitamin A was most commonly measured in international units (IU), including on the Nutrition Facts label. However, the Institute of Medicine (2001) lists RDA of vitamin A in micrograms (mcg) of retinol activity equivalents (RAE) to account for the different absorption rates of preformed vitamin A and provitamin A carotenoids. Under the Food and Drug Administration's (FDA) new food and dietary supplement labeling regulations, as of July 2018 large companies may no longer list vitamin A in IU but instead must list units in mcg RAE. Table 6.11 highlights the RDA and UL for vitamin A as well as foods rich in the nutrient.

TABLE 6.11   Vitamin A: Intake Guidelines and Food Sources

RDA	Males ages 19 and up: 900 mcg RAE (equivalent to 3,000 IU)
	Females ages 19 and up: 700 mcg RAE (equivalent to 2,333 IU)
UL	3,000 mcg (equivalent to 10,000 IU).
Foods rich in vitamin A	Leafy green vegetables (kale, spinach, broccoli), orange and yellow vegetables (carrots, sweet potatoes, pumpkin and other winter squash, summer squash), tomatoes, red bell pepper, cantaloupe, mango, beef liver, fish oils, milk, eggs

Data from: National Institutes of Health Office of Dietary Supplments; Available: https://ods.od.nih.gov/Health-Information/nutrientrecommendations.aspx. Data from: Harvard T.H. Chan School of Public Health; Available: https://www.hsph.harvard.edu/nutritionsource/.

Zeaxanthin and Lutein: Keys to Better Vision?

In the context of sport performance it is important to briefly discuss zeaxanthin and lutein, two carotenoids found in high concentrations in the human eye; these are closely related to vitamin A but are unable to be converted into retinol. Products that supplement these two carotenoids are becoming increasingly popular, especially among athletes who rely on their visual acuity. Pitchers in baseball, football players in skill-based positions, and even race car drivers have begun using these supplements for potential improvements like increased visual acuity and color contrast, reduced sensitivity to light and glare, reduced dryness and irritation, and improved reaction speed. It is also well researched at this point that consistent intake of zeaxanthin and lutein can protect against the harmful effects of blue light, to which young athletes in particular are exposed in high volume. A review by Renzi-Hammond and colleagues (2017) indicates that the athletes who would see the most benefit from supplements are those who are not consuming enough zeaxanthin and lutein in their diet. Some foods that are rich in these nutrients are leafy green vegetables, orange and yellow fruits and vegetables, corn, eggs, and broccoli. Most zeaxanthin and lutein products offer somewhere between 20 and 40 milligrams of the two components combined. There is no RDA for them specifically.

Vitamin D (Calciferol)

Vitamin D is commonly associated with bone health but is wildly important for many other processes. Vitamin D promotes calcium absorption in the gut and acts as a buffer for maintaining calcium levels in the blood. Vitamin D and calcium (discussed later in the chapter) frequently work in tandem, which is why you often see them in supplements together. Together with calcium, vitamin D helps protect against osteoporosis. Without sufficient vitamin D, bones can become thin and brittle. Vitamin D also plays a role in managing inflammation and moderating cell growth as well as in neuromuscular and immune function, genome modulation, and glucose metabolism, specifically with the role of insulin secretion and sensitivity. In foods and dietary supplements, vitamin D has two main forms, D_2 (ergocalciferol) and D_3 (cholecalciferol). Both forms are well absorbed. The presence of fat in the gut enhances vitamin D absorption, but some vitamin D is absorbed even without dietary fat.

Few foods naturally contain vitamin D; in the United States fortified foods provide most of the vitamin D in people's diets. It is commonly available as a dietary supplement. It is also produced by the body when ultraviolet (UV) rays from sunlight are absorbed through the skin and trigger vitamin D synthesis—this is the most bioavailable form of vitamin D.

Vitamin D deficiency is common and well documented at this point in time. Some groups are at higher risk for vitamin D deficiency, including older adults (perhaps as a result of more time spent indoors or a limited ability of older skin to synthesize vitamin D), those who live at or north of 42 degrees latitude (northern United States and Canada), and individuals with darker skin pigmentation (which is less efficient at synthesizing vitamin D from sunlight). From an athletic standpoint, athletes who spend most of their time indoors or wear uniforms that cover a lot of their skin when they're outside should also be considered higher risk for deficiency. Similarly, athletes who have a dairy allergy or lactose intolerance may be more susceptible to deficiency because of a limited ability to include foods rich in vitamin D in their diet.

Many vitamin D supplements provide well in excess of the UL, so it's important to not take high doses of supplements if you are not deficient. In excess, vitamin D interferes with calcium metabolism and can cause very high levels of calcium in the blood. This can cause vomiting, diarrhea, and even kidney failure. Additionally, excessively high levels of vitamin D actually lower the bioavailable forms of vitamin D in your blood and can lead to increased risk of fractures (Sanders, Nicholson, and Ebeling 2012). Table 6.12 highlights the RDA and UL for vitamin D as well as foods rich in the nutrient.

TABLE 6.12   **Vitamin D: Intake Guidelines and Food Sources**

RDA	Males and females ages 19-70: 15 mcg (600 IU)
UL	4,000 IU
Foods rich in vitamin D	Cod liver oil, rainbow trout, salmon (sockeye), mushrooms treated with UV, fortified milk, fortified soy, almond and oat milks, fortified ready-to-eat cereal, sardines, eggs (whole), beef liver, tuna fish, cheddar cheese

Data from: National Institutes of Health Office of Dietary Supplments; Available: https://ods.od.nih.gov/Health-Information/nutrientrecommendations.aspx. Data from: Harvard T.H. Chan School of Public Health; Available: https://www.hsph.harvard.edu/nutritionsource/.

Vitamin E

Vitamin E is the collective name for a group of naturally occurring compounds called *tocopherols* and *tocotrienols*. Vitamin E exists in eight chemical forms, but alpha-tocopherol is the only form that is recognized to meet human requirements.

Vitamin E primarily functions as an antioxidant. As mentioned previously, antioxidants protect cells from the damaging effects of free radicals. Although free radicals are a natural byproduct of normal bodily functions, excessive production of them can lead to oxidative stress and damage to other cells and are thought to contribute to the development of cardiovascular disease and some cancers. The body is also exposed to free radicals from environmental exposures, such as cigarette smoke, air pollution, and ultraviolet radiation. Although research is still not conclusive, it's thought that antioxidants such as vitamin E might help prevent or delay the chronic diseases associated with free radicals; however, this is hard to study definitively because of the sheer number of antioxidants.

In addition to its activities as an antioxidant, vitamin E is involved in immune function and many other metabolic processes. For athletes, sufficient levels of vitamin E may be key in helping manage inflammation, which can be elevated during high training loads or if training at altitude or in extreme climates (Jiang 2014). However, further research is needed to assess whether vitamin E supplementation past the RDA may be beneficial for athletes.

Supplements of vitamin E typically provide only alpha-tocopherol, although products containing other tocopherols and even tocotrienols are available. Most vitamin E–only supplements provide amounts substantially higher than the RDA. As discussed before, a multivitamin is likely the best approach to fill in any nutritional gaps without getting any one nutrient in excess. Table 6.13 highlights the RDA and UL for vitamin E as well as foods rich in the nutrient. Vitamin E recommendations are for alpha-tocopherol alone, the only form maintained in plasma.

TABLE 6.13   Vitamin E: Intake Guidelines and Food Sources

RDA	Males and females ages 14 and up: 15 mg (22.4 IU)
UL	1,000 mg (1,500 IU)
Foods rich in vitamin E	Soybean, canola, sunflower, safflower, corn, and wheat germ oils; dry roasted sunflower seeds, almonds, and peanuts; hazelnuts; peanut butter; spinach; kiwi; mango; broccoli (cooked); tomato (raw)

Data from: National Institutes of Health Office of Dietary Supplments; Available: https://ods.od.nih.gov/Health-Information/nutrientrecommendations.aspx. Data from: Harvard T.H. Chan School of Public Health; Available: https://www.hsph.harvard.edu/nutritionsource/.

Vitamin K

Vitamin K includes vitamin K_1, which is found mostly in green leafy vegetables and is the main form of vitamin K in the human diet, and vitamin K_2, which can be found in small amounts in some animal-based and fermented foods and can also be produced in the gut.

Vitamin K is a necessary coenzyme involved in the processes of blood clotting and bone metabolism, as well as other important physiological functions. Like other fat-soluble vitamins, vitamin K absorption is improved when there is dietary fat present. Vitamin K is usually not assessed unless a person takes anticoagulants or has a specific bleeding disorder.

The interrelationships between vitamin K, estrogen, and bone metabolism may be of interest to athletes, although more research is needed in this area—despite hypotheses by Braam and colleagues (2003) that vitamin K supplementation may help prevent or reverse loss in bone mineral density in athletic populations, they found no difference in the study and placebo groups. Getting sufficient amounts of vitamin K is important and can help promote good bone health. Deficiency is more common than once thought, so athletes should strive to include adequate amounts in their diet or via a multivitamin. Because research is inadequate to support creating an RDA for vitamin K, there is instead an established AI. Table 6.14 highlights the AI and UL for vitamin K as well as foods rich in the nutrient.

TABLE 6.14   Vitamin K: Intake Guidelines and Food Sources

AI	Males ages 19 and up: 120 mcg Females ages 19 and up: 90 mcg
UL	None
Foods rich in vitamin K	Spinach, collard greens, turnip greens, kale, broccoli, iceberg lettuce, soybean oil, canola oil, edamame

Data from: National Institutes of Health Office of Dietary Supplments; Available: https://ods.od.nih.gov/Health-Information/nutrientrecommendations.aspx. Data from: Harvard T.H. Chan School of Public Health; Available: https://www.hsph.harvard.edu/nutritionsource/.

Minerals

Minerals are elements that our bodies need to grow and function normally. There are 20 minerals that are considered essential for the body, many of which are particularly important for athletes. The following sections will cover the ones most pertinent to sport.

Calcium

Calcium is perhaps best known for making up much of the structure of our bones and teeth. However, it has many other functions, including helping to control blood vessel function, muscle contraction, blood clotting, and nerve and hormone regulation. The absorption of calcium is hardwired to ebb and flow depending on how much the body needs at that time. If you are taking in high amounts of calcium your body will naturally absorb a smaller percentage to help prevent getting too much in your system; conversely, if you're not getting adequate amounts of calcium your body will enhance absorption in an effort to make sure that you're getting enough. Calcium absorption can also be affected by age.

The amount of calcium absorbed also varies by food source. Certain compounds in plants decrease calcium absorption by forming compounds that are not digestible. Because of this, absorption of calcium from a food like spinach is only around 5 percent, whereas in a food like milk it is much higher—nearly 30 percent. As discussed previously, vitamin D also acts synergistically with calcium. Low levels of vitamin D can lead to decreased calcium absorption, which can ultimately affect bone health and calcium balance in the body.

Although critical for anyone, athletes should be especially attuned to their bone health, given that exercise and bone health are closely related and that the risk of bone injury bears heavy on an athlete's mind. Humans are only able to build bone until their early to mid 20s, so it is critical to have good habits in place to help maximize bone building and reduce bone loss. Things that help build bone include weight-bearing exercise, proper hormonal activity, and adequate nutrients like calcium and vitamin D. As with so many aspects of diet, aiming for a variety of different foods within each food group helps to ensure adequate amounts of these nutrients. Table 6.15 highlights the RDA and UL for calcium as well as foods rich in the nutrient.

Potassium

Potassium is vital for maintaining fluid volume in the body and has a direct relationship with sodium, which also regulates fluid volume in

TABLE 6.15   Calcium: Intake Guidelines and Food Sources

RDA	Males ages 19-70: 1,000 mg Males ages 71 and up: 1,200 mg Females ages 19-50: 1,000 mg Females ages 51 and up: 1,200 mg
UL	2,500 mg
Foods rich in calcium	Yogurt, milk, mozzarella cheese, cottage cheese, soft serve ice cream, tofu, soybeans, canned salmon or sardines with bones, chia seeds, leafy greens (spinach, turnip greens, kale, bok choy), foods fortified with calcium (e.g., breakfast cereal, soy milk, orange juice)

Data from: National Institutes of Health Office of Dietary Supplments; Available: https://ods.od.nih.gov/Health-Information/nutrientrecommendations.aspx. Data from: Harvard T.H. Chan School of Public Health; Available: https://www.hsph.harvard.edu/nutritionsource/.

the body. It is uncommon to assess potassium status, because getting an accurate result is difficult; most potassium within the body is stored inside the cells and not within the bloodstream.

The body absorbs potassium well—around 85 to 90 percent, potentially even higher if potassium stores in the body are low. It's important to get potassium from your diet daily, and luckily, it's found in a number of common foods and beverages. Because research is inadequate to support creating an RDA for potassium, there is instead an established AI for all ages based on the highest median potassium intakes in healthy adults. Table 6.16 highlights the AI and UL for potassium as well as foods rich in the nutrient.

TABLE 6.16   Potassium: Intake Guidelines and Food Sources

AI*	Males: 3,400 mg Females: 2,600 mg
UL	None
Foods rich in potassium	Apricots (dried), prunes, raisins, lentils, acorn squash, potato (skin on), kidney beans, orange juice, soybeans, bananas, milk, spinach, chicken breast, yogurt (plain or Greek), salmon, beef, molasses, tomatoes, soy milk, broccoli, cantaloupe, turkey breast, asparagus, apple (skin on), cashews, brown rice, tuna (canned)

*AIs do not apply to individuals with impaired potassium excretion because of medical conditions (e.g., kidney disease) or the use of medications that impair potassium excretion.

Data from: National Institutes of Health Office of Dietary Supplments; Available: https://ods.od.nih.gov/Health-Information/nutrientrecommendations.aspx. Data from: Harvard T.H. Chan School of Public Health; Available: https://www.hsph.harvard.edu/nutritionsource/.

Sodium

Like potassium, sodium is an electrolyte, which are minerals in the body that carry an electric charge and are essential for various bodily functions. Sodium and potassium are very much interconnected—both are essential nutrients and play key roles in maintaining fluid balance—but they actually have opposite effects in the body. Whereas sodium intake increases blood pressure, potassium intake can actually help relax blood vessels while decreasing blood pressure. Our bodies require significantly more potassium than sodium each day; however, typical intake is the opposite.

Sodium is commonly found in sodium chloride, most commonly known as table salt, which is made up of around 40 percent sodium and 60 percent chloride. The human body needs a small amount of sodium to help maintain fluid balance, as well as control nerve impulses and regulate muscle contractions. Although this small amount is vital, it is not a nutrient that is hard to come by because it is so commonly used in food flavorings and preservatives. In fact, most adults (especially in developed countries) have a hard time controlling sodium intake, which in high amounts can lead to high blood pressure and subsequent negative health outcomes. Although salting your food can contribute to increased

A Salty Question

A common misconception about salt is that some kinds are better for you than others. Despite differences in color, origin, and crystal size, however, there are few significant differences between types of salt. Although some salts, like the currently popular pink Himalayan sea salt, do have some minerals in them that refined table salt does not, the amounts are negligible—especially considering that total salt intake should generally be limited. Crystal size can also make a difference in how much salt ends up on your food (finer salt may lend itself to using more overall), but the actual salt itself is no different.

Ironically, table salt—specifically, iodized table salt—may be the healthiest choice you can make when it comes to salt in your diet. Many decades ago, it became common practice to fortify table salt with iodine, a necessary nutrient that American diets in particular tend to lack. Iodine plays a vital role in the production of thyroid hormones, which regulate metabolism, growth, and development, and deficiency can lead to serious health concerns (most notoriously, goiter, an abnormal enlargement of the thyroid gland). Iodized table salt is a great way to ensure adequate iodine intake.

sodium intake, for most people this does not come close to the amount eaten via commercially prepared, packaged, and processed foods, which comprise the vast majority of the sodium in our diets.

It's important for athletes specifically to be purposeful about sodium intake. Because sodium is the primary electrolyte lost in sweat, athletes likely need higher amounts of sodium than their nonathlete counterparts, particularly if they are very heavy sweaters or tend to eat very fresh, minimally processed foods. For this reason, I often recommend that athletes focus on sodium-rich beverages or products when hydrating, as opposed to sports drinks that contain mostly potassium and little to no sodium, which do not address the primary electrolyte lost. However, if you struggle to control symptoms like cramping, then you may find it helpful to add a moderate amount of potassium as well. The exact amount of sodium lost in sweat depends not only on how much sweat is lost during a workout, but also on your individual propensity to lose sodium in your sweat. Ultimately this number is unique and requires sweat testing to quantify. Some sweat tests will also measure potassium loss, but more as a measure for accuracy as opposed to an objective measure to aid replacement. Details about sweat testing and more recommendations for hydration are discussed in chapter 7.

Regardless of your individual sodium losses, I recommend thinking about your sodium intake in a periodized fashion. When you're four or more hours from training or competition, try to choose mostly minimally processed foods that are low in sodium, such as fruit, vegetables, whole grains, nuts, meat, and dairy. As training approaches you can start to think about including more sodium, especially if you are a heavy sweater, have had issues with cramping, or if it's expected to be an especially hot or humid environment for training. This may mean salting your food, choosing salty snacks like pretzels or crackers, or having a sports drink that contains sodium.

It is important to remember, however, that excess sodium over time can contribute to increased blood pressure and other health complications. Although this isn't generally a concern for young, healthy athletes, it's important to keep in mind as you progress through your career and eventually transition out. If you're not consistently working up a sweat—whether it's the off-season, you're injured, your level of competition has decreased, or you've retired from sport—you should look to discontinue the use of high sodium supplements and from going too wild with the table salt at meals. The practice of purposefully including more sodium only around periods of intense training and subsequent heavy sweating can help promote good long-term health, but too much sodium otherwise can lead to various health complications over time. Table 6.17 highlights the AI and UL for sodium as well as foods rich in the nutrient.

TABLE 6.17   Sodium: Intake Guidelines and Food Sources

AI	Males and females ages 14 and up: 1,500 mg
UL	None; however, due to the risk of long-term high intake, a chronic disease risk reduction (CDRR) intake has been established at 2,300 mg
Foods high in sodium	Soup, salty snacks (chips, crackers, pretzels, popcorn), deli meats and cheeses, breads, canned beans and vegetables, frozen dinners and pizza

Data from: National Institutes of Health Office of Dietary Supplments; Available: https://ods.od.nih.gov/Health-Information/nutrientrecommendations.aspx. Data from: Harvard T.H. Chan School of Public Health; Available: https://www.hsph.harvard.edu/nutritionsource/.

Iron

Iron is an essential component of hemoglobin, a protein in red blood cells that transfers oxygen from the lungs to other tissues in the body. Although this oxygen delivery is what garners the most attention, iron is also an integral component of muscle and soft-tissue metabolism, physical growth and brain development, and the synthesis of certain hormones.

When discussing dietary iron it's important to distinguish between the two forms: heme and nonheme. Heme iron is found in animal sources like meat and seafood, whereas nonheme is found in plant sources like leafy greens, grains, and legumes. The notable difference between the two is that heme iron is far more bioavailable than nonheme, meaning that you need to eat much more nonheme iron to absorb the same amount that you could get from a much smaller amount of heme iron.

Although all humans need iron, certain populations are at higher risk for having low iron. Females are at higher risk due to blood loss via menses, and endurance runners are also at a higher risk due to iron lost in red blood cell breakdown that happens as their feet hit the ground (a phenomena called *foot strike hemolysis*). Reliable iron assessment requires a blood draw. However, because this analysis may be affected by inflammation, it's important to get tested during a low training time frame or on an off day.

Table 6.18 highlights the RDA and UL for iron as well as foods rich in the nutrient. When choosing iron-rich foods it's important to remember the difference in bioavailability between animal and plant sources; animal sources (heme iron) will be absorbed much better by the body that plant-based sources (nonheme iron).

Magnesium

Magnesium is involved in over 300 enzymatic reactions in the body that regulate everything from protein synthesis to muscle and nerve function to blood pressure and blood sugar regulation. It's an integral

TABLE 6.18   Iron: Intake Guidelines and Food Sources

RDA*	Males and postmenopausal females: 8 mg Menstrual females: 18 mg
UL	45 mg
Foods rich in iron	Breakfast cereals, kidney beans, white beans, broccoli, spinach, lentils, chickpeas, pistachios, tofu, rice (white and brown), bread (whole-wheat and white), whole-wheat pasta, potatoes (skin on), dark chocolate, oysters, sardines (canned), beef liver, poultry, tuna, eggs

*RDA given is for nonvegetarians; the RDA for vegetarians is 1.8 times higher due to the difference in bioavailability between plant and animal sources.

Data from: National Institutes of Health Office of Dietary Supplments; Available: https://ods.od.nih.gov/Health-Information/nutrientrecommendations.aspx. Data from: Harvard T.H. Chan School of Public Health; Available: https://www.hsph.harvard.edu/nutritionsource/.

component of carbohydrate metabolism, as well as a required nutrient in the formation of bone. Magnesium also plays a role in the transport of calcium and potassium across cell membranes, a process that is important for muscle contraction and ensures a normal heart rhythm. Magnesium can be lost in sweat, but the amount is negligible and should not be supplemented specifically with the purpose of replacing these trace amounts.

Definitive research does not currently show magnesium to have an ergogenic effect on athletic performance, but some research has started to show promising effects. One study by Reno and colleagues (2022) found that 350 milligrams of magnesium supplementation for 10 days significantly reduced muscle soreness, though the majority of participants appeared to have low dietary magnesium intake upon baseline. Another area of interest around magnesium supplementation has been its role in helping to promote sleep. A review by Arab and colleagues (2022) found that in observational studies, magnesium supplementation was linked to better sleep quality, though more long-term, well-controlled studies are needed. Anecdotally, however, many athletes feel that magnesium helps improve their sleep, and in reasonable doses it could be a low-risk way to help promote good sleep and abate muscle soreness for athletes.

Table 6.19 highlights the AI and UL for magnesium as well as foods rich in the nutrient.

Zinc

Zinc is an essential mineral that is involved in hundreds of enzymatic reactions. It is essential in DNA synthesis and wound healing, and in relation to athletic performance, zinc is very involved with MPS. A study by Kilic and colleagues (2006) found that zinc supplementation may also

TABLE 6.19   Magnesium: Intake Guidelines and Food Sources

AI	Males ages 19-30: 400 mg Males ages 31 and up: 420 mg Females ages 19-30: 310 mg Females ages 31 and up: 320 mg
UL	350 mg; higher doses can lead to diarrhea, nausea, and cramping
Foods rich in magnesium	Pumpkin seeds, chia seeds, almonds, peanuts, cashews, raisins, avocados, bananas, spinach (cooked), soy milk, black beans, edamame, peanut butter, potato (skin on), brown rice, yogurt, milk, salmon, chicken breast, oatmeal, fortified breakfast cereals

Data from: National Institutes of Health Office of Dietary Supplments; Available: https://ods.od.nih.gov/factsheets/Magnesium-HealthProfessional/.

prevent the decrease in thyroid hormones and testosterone that comes along with exhaustive exercise—which, given the role that testosterone plays in muscle synthesis, suggests that adequate zinc levels may help promote building lean muscle mass.

It is also well established that zinc plays an important role in immune health. Wessels, Maywald, and Rink (2017) note that zinc homeostasis (i.e., not having too much or too little) is crucial for defending the body from invading pathogens as well as protecting the body from an overactive immune system. For this reason, ensuring sufficient intake of zinc—either through a well-balanced diet or supplementation—is important for athletes to support performance, recovery, and overall health. However, research does not currently support needs above the RDA for athletes. Table 6.20 highlights the RDA and UL for zinc as well as foods rich in the nutrient.

TABLE 6.20   Zinc: Intake Guidelines and Food Sources

RDA	Males ages 19 and up: 11 mg Females ages 19 and up: 8 mg
UL	40 mg
Foods rich in zinc	Shellfish, pork, beef, poultry, legumes, nuts, seeds, whole grains, fortified breakfast cereals

Data from: National Institutes of Health Office of Dietary Supplments; Available: https://www.hsph.harvard.edu/nutritionsource/zinc/.

The roles of vitamins and minerals in the human body are vast. In many cases the need for these micronutrients is elevated further for athletes who are pushing their bodies to physical limits. It's important for athletes to ensure they meet their recommended daily intake of vitamins and minerals through a well-balanced diet that includes a variety of nutrient-rich foods in order to optimize exercise performance, enhance endurance, and reduce the risk of fatigue and injury. In some cases, supplementation may be necessary, but this should be done under the guidance of a registered dietitian to avoid excessive intake or interactions with medications, and care should be taken to ensure that you are choosing a quality product. More information on how to approach supplements can be found in chapter 8. Ultimately, proper nutrition with an emphasis on vitamins and minerals is essential for athletes to support their performance and overall health and well-being.

CHAPTER 7
Sustain High Performance With Hydration

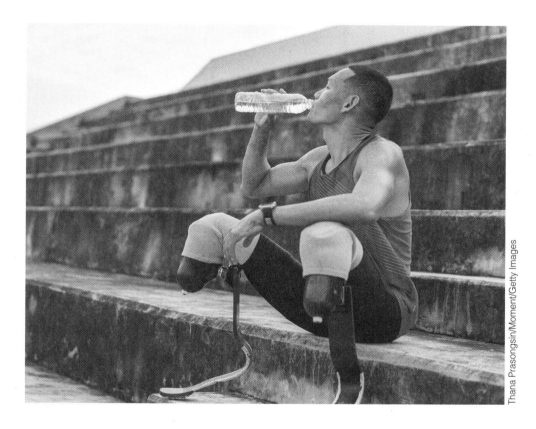

Thana Prasongsin/Moment/Getty Images

The human body comprises roughly 60 to 70 percent water, and it is crucial for nearly every bodily process. Water helps regulate body temperature, excrete waste, moisten bodily tissues, protect organs, lubricate joints, and deliver nutrients to various bodily systems. Proper hydration is therefore vital to ensure that these processes run as seamlessly as possible. Many athletes are generally aware that hydration is important, but far fewer recognize just how important, and how timing can play into what liquids—and how much of them—to choose when.

During exercise, fluid is lost a few different ways. Most people think of sweat, which is often the biggest contributor to fluid loss during exercise. Sweat helps cool the body by getting the skin wet and taking heat with it when it evaporates. However, you are also losing fluid via respiration, and of course, through normal bodily functions as well: in your GI tract to help turn food into digestible nutrients, as well by your kidneys and other organs for urine production. Although these things occur during any activity, it should come as no surprise that environment is hugely influential. A hotter, more humid environment will promote more sweat loss, whereas a cold environment increases water lost through respiration. The latter effect is slight, but if you are practicing outside for hours per day, or even just spending a lot of time outside, this effect could add up!

Fluid Needs

One of the most common questions I get asked is, "How much fluid do I need?" Although the question seems simple, the answer is not. The amount of fluid an individual needs depends on a number of factors, including sex, body size, and the propensity to sweat—the last of which is arguably the most important. Most athletes can picture the teammate whose shirt is drenched after every practice and the teammate who did the same exact workout and has hardly lost a drop of sweat. This simply boils down to the individual athlete's propensity to sweat. Although there

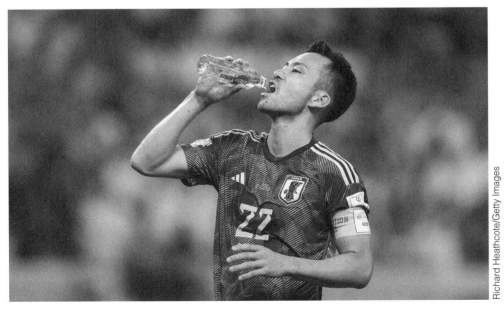

Richard Heathcote/Getty Images

Individualizing your hydration plan is important for not only your health but also your performance.

is some speculation that individuals who are highly trained may sweat less as a result of better conditioning, there is not good evidence that this is the case.

Other hugely influential factors include the environment in which you exercise (heat, humidity), your clothing, your physical fitness level, and the intensity and duration of the activity itself. Not surprisingly, the hotter and more humid the environment, the more an athlete will tend to sweat (figure 7.1). Similarly, a uniform made of heavier material and covering more surface area will cause athletes to sweat more. A football player wearing pads, pants, and a helmet is likely to sweat considerably more than a cross country runner wearing a tank top and short shorts.

As you can imagine, it can be difficult to make a fluid recommendation without considering these different factors. However, there are

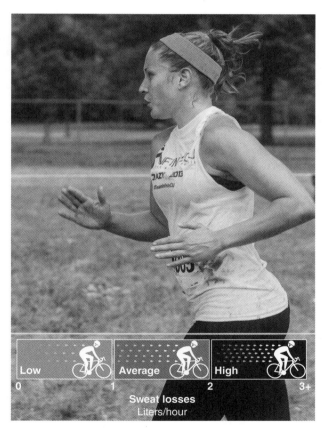

FIGURE 7.1   Exercising in extreme heat and humidity greatly affects your sweat rate, so remember to adjust your hydration intake accordingly.

Reprinted by permission from B. Murray and W.L. Kenney, *Practical Guide to Exercise Physiology,* (Champaign, IL: Human Kinetics, 2016), 67.

some general recommendations that can function as a starting point: One common suggestion is to consume 0.5 to 1 fluid ounce per pound of body weight.

From the most basic standpoint, one of the easiest ways to assess hydration status is to look at the color of your urine when you go to the bathroom. Urine does not need to be clear but should be light yellow, like lemonade. If your urine is dark yellow or brownish (like apple juice), that is a sign that you need to step up your hydration game.

Dehydration

Dehydration, or the state of inadequate hydration, can be extremely detrimental to performance. As noted by Sawka (1992), dehydration reduces the amount of blood pumped by your heart to the rest of your body during exercise, especially in the heat—meaning that exercise is physiologically harder when not hydrated. Dehydration of 2 percent or more of your body weight—for example, a 200-pound athlete losing 4 pounds—negatively affects practically every aspect of performance, both physically and mentally. Adan (2012) mentions that a 2 percent fluid deficit impairs performance in tasks that require attention, psychomotor, and immediate memory skills. Perhaps the biggest difference between hydration and other nutrition habits is that the negative effects seen from dehydration are almost immediate. Although many poor nutrition habits might catch up with you over time, lack of proper hydration affects you that same day. Symptoms of dehydration include the following:

Increased thirst

Dry mouth and throat

Dark yellow or amber-colored urine

Muscle cramps

Fatigue and weakness

Dizziness or lightheadedness

Loss of appetite

Headache

You should stop and seek medical attention if you experience any of the following symptoms of severe dehydration:

Decreased urine output

Rapid heartbeat

Sunken eyes

Confusion or irritability

Fainting

Excessive Hydration

Although hydration is very important, your consumption during exercise should not exceed your sweat losses. Not only can excessive fluid cause GI discomfort, but drinking excessive water can put you at risk for developing hyponatremia, a very serious condition that occurs when sodium levels are too low. The population most at risk for hyponatremia are athletes participating in ultraendurance activities who are only replacing sweat losses with water. Hew-Butler and colleagues (2015) recommend for ultraendurance athletes to drink to thirst when possible, but to understand their individual fluid needs and ensure that sodium-containing foods and beverages are made available during training and competition.

Mild cases of hyponatremia may not cause noticeable symptoms, but as the condition worsens symptoms may include nausea, headache, confusion, fatigue, muscle weakness and cramps, seizures, and in the most severe cases even coma and death. Treatment depends on the severity of the condition. For a milder case, increasing dietary sodium or decreasing fluid intake (or both) may be sufficient. If more severe, intravenous saline solutions or medications may be necessary. Severe symptoms of hyponatremia should be treated as a medical emergency.

Fluid Intake Timing

Similar to other nutrients we've discussed thus far, water also has some important considerations regarding timing around your workouts: Approaching hydration purposefully can help maximize training and promote good performance. The following recommendations will help you time your hydration before, during, and after training or competition.

Before the Workout

You should ultimately aim to be adequately hydrated when heading into training or competition—last-minute attempts to drink after not hydrating all day are futile. Sawka and colleagues (2007) recommend drinking 5 to 7 milliliters per kilogram of body weight at least four hours before exercise and, if needed, 3 to 5 milliliters per kilogram of body weight two hours before exercise. Goulet (2012) states that endurance athletes specifically should aim to start exercise well hydrated, which can be achieved by keeping thirst sensation low and urine color pale and by drinking approximately 5 to 10 milliliters per kilogram of body weight of water two hours before exercise.

During the Workout

During training, it's generally recommended to drink every 15 to 20 minutes, especially if it's hot or humid. However, many athletes must rely on their coaches to provide breaks with that frequency. If your coach does not, you might consider talking to them about the importance of hydration in terms of health and performance. If they are still reluctant to give frequent breaks, or if the environment for any reason makes it hard to do so, make sure to maximize your intake at breaks you do get. If it is especially hot or humid or if breaks are limited. you may not be able to afford to just sip water. Although you don't want to chug fluid and upset your stomach, you can try to take gulps to ensure you're getting enough.

Some other practical considerations can also be the temperature of the fluid: Most people enjoy colder fluids when it's warm, but if it's so cold that it's hard to drink quickly you may be deterred from getting enough. Additionally, if you dislike water, consider using a sports drink or even flavored water if needed. Anything that can help increase total fluid intake is a positive and ensures hydration.

After the Workout

Even after you finish your training session or competition, hydration doesn't stop! I recommend that athletes continue to sip fluids for the hour or two after finishing exercise—keep in mind that the body only absorbs fluid at a certain rate, so there is no need to chug a bunch of fluid all at once. You can aim to drink until your thirst is quenched, plus a little bit more, or more specifically 2 to 3 cups (16-24 fl oz) of fluid per pound that you lost during exercise (using weight to determine fluid losses will be discussed in the next section). Keep in mind too that your postworkout beverage choices encompass more than just water—by choosing a beverage like a protein shake or chocolate milk you can hydrate *and* support recovery needs.

Individualizing Your Plan

Beyond the general recommendations, you may need to individualize your hydration plan a bit further. If your urine is consistently light in color and you do not have any specific problems with staying hydrated there is no reason for you to test more specifically. However, if you are experiencing symptoms of dehydration (cramping, fatigue, headaches, etc.) and feel that you could benefit from knowing more details about your hydration needs you might consider some of the following tests.

Weighing In and Out

Weighing yourself before and immediately after a workout is one of the simplest ways to assess fluid loss. It is a common misconception by athletes that weight loss during a workout is true weight from fat. The practice of wearing sweats to try to promote sweating to "get weight down" is an old-school favorite that unfortunately is doing nothing besides causing dehydration. It is well documented that even during longer workouts of two to four hours, any weight that is lost is not coming from fat or muscle mass, but instead from fluid. Small amounts of fat and muscle loss have been seen during ultraendurance training of six to eight hours or more (Knechtle, Rosemann, and Nikolaidis 2018), but most athletes should assume that any weight loss during a workout is simply from fluid.

With this in mind, measuring your pre- and postworkout weight will help you easily quantify fluid loss. It's important to take both weights wearing the same clothes and shoes so as not to skew the results based on equipment. If you are a swimmer, you should shower prior to the initial weigh-in so that you simulate similar conditions that will be present when you get out of the pool afterward.

As mentioned previously, it is recommended to drink 2 to 3 cups (16-24 fl oz) of fluid per pound lost. Once you have determined how many pounds you lost, you should aim to replace that fluid over the next four to six hours. Therefore, an athlete who lost 5 pounds during a workout or competition should aim to drink 10 to 15 cups of fluid over the four to six hours following the conclusion of that workout. In the case of extreme fluid loss this time frame may not be realistic, but you will want to ensure that you have replaced that fluid before your next workout. Although replacing lost fluids is paramount, if you are consistently losing a fair amount of weight during training you should also focus on consuming more fluids throughout training to minimize these losses.

For most athletes, the simple practice of weighing in and weighing out a couple of times is more than enough to help guide hydration without creating too much of a focus on body weight. Getting a general feel for how much weight you tend to lose during certain types of training will give you a good goal to aim for in terms of rehydrating. However, as mentioned throughout this book, if you have struggled with body image or if weighing yourself causes you stress and anxiety, this practice is probably not in your best interest. You would likely be better off monitoring your urine color, and as long as you are not a very heavy sweater and not having problems staying hydrated, this should be adequate.

Sweat Rate Testing

Sweat rate testing builds off this weighing in and out practice to calculate your individual sweat rate, or the amount of fluid you lose per hour via sweat. This is more involved and requires a fair amount of control of your environment immediately around the workout. In addition to weighing in and out, you also need to track any fluids in and out of your body. This includes total ounces consumed from your water bottle, as well as volume of urine output, if applicable. There are great sweat rate calculators online—a quick search should yield many options that allow you to hone in on this aspect of your performance.

Sweat Testing

Objectively evaluating hydration status via formal sweat testing involves not only measuring sweat rate, as outlined previously, but also includes wearing patches to collect sweat so that you can quantify the amount of electrolytes (specifically sodium) that are being lost. Although sweat testing has historically been limited to high-level athletes working with practitioners who have access to labs, accessibility has increased substantially in recent years with the development of sweat patches that can be used even by the layperson. Purchased online or through local sporting goods stores, these patches are worn during a training session or competition and used in conjunction with an app to measure sweat rate and the amount of electrolytes lost. If you do use one of these sweat tests, I would encourage you to try to do them in a controlled environment for the best possible results and to pay close attention to those results. Most of these tests will not only tell you your individual sweat information, but also suggest changes you could make to improve your hydration habits based on those results.

As a reminder, all of these methods for assessing your hydration status can be helpful, but none are necessary for the majority of athletes. If you are managing your hydration well (urine is generally light colored and you have no cramping, unusual levels of fatigue, lightheadedness, or overheating) then there is generally no need to delve further into these specifics. However, if you are struggling with hydration in any manner, one of these tests can help you better manage this aspect of your fueling.

Types of Hydration

Now that you've learned how to determine how much fluid you might need, it's important to discuss what types of fluid you should be choosing. Many people assume that water is the only good choice and that any other beverage might be detrimental. In fact, most beverages are hydrating and can be included as part of a solid hydration plan (see figure 7.2)—including flavored water, 100 percent fruit or veggie juice, milk or milk alternatives, protein shakes, sports drinks, and even tea and coffee. There is a common misconception that coffee does not contribute to hydration efforts or even that it is actively dehydrating via a diuretic effect. However, in moderation coffee does not have a diuretic effect—the caffeine in coffee acts as a stimulant, which also stimulates the bladder. So even though coffee may make you have to pee, it only affects the water that is already processed and in your bladder, and as long as it's consumed in reasonable amounts (less than 4 cups of regular coffee per day) there is no need for concern.

From a hydration and performance standpoint, the only beverages I recommend you limit (especially immediately around activity) are energy drinks, soda, and drinks made with full-fat dairy like whole milk or cream. Energy drinks are concerning because most are not well-regulated and it can be difficult to know exactly how much caffeine is in them; this will be discussed in more depth in chapter 8. Although soda tends to have a lot of sugar (aka quick carbohydrates), the carbonation tends to not be ideal for most athletes and can cause GI upset, which can be exacerbated by the artificial sweeteners in some sodas. Full-fat dairy (either on their own or included in tasty coffee drinks) have a high protein and fat content and can also cause GI distress and unfavorable GI symptoms if consumed too close to activity.

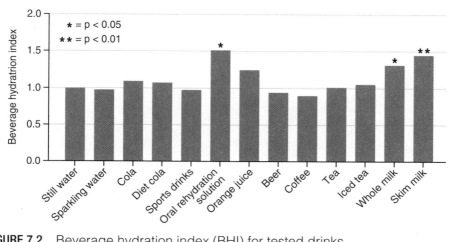

FIGURE 7.2 Beverage hydration index (BHI) for tested drinks.

Electrolytes

For many athletes, drinking the appropriate amount of fluids is sufficient to manage hydration and avoid symptoms associated with dehydration. However, athletes who are especially heavy sweaters or have a history of muscle cramps should also pay close attention to their intake of electrolytes. Electrolytes refer to a handful of essential minerals that are vital for many bodily functions, but in this context they are specifically key in maintaining fluid balance. Having a fluid imbalance between tissues is what can lead to dehydration, fatigue, and muscle cramps. The notable electrolytes that pertain to hydration are sodium, potassium, magnesium, and calcium, all of which are outlined more in depth in chapter 6. Although potassium has gained some popularity in sports drinks and in the general realm of hydration as of late, it's vital to understand that the primary electrolyte lost in sweat is sodium.

Although there's no objective way to define whether or not you are a heavy sweater, if you notice your clothes and hair are very wet after exercise or find that you lose a significant amount of weight, you are likely a heavy sweater. You may also be a salty sweater, meaning that you lose high amounts of electrolytes in your sweat. In addition to doing formal sweat testing, salty sweaters can sometimes self-identify by paying

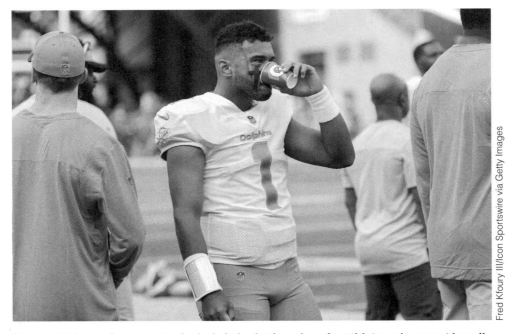

Fred Kfoury III/Icon Sportswire via Getty Images

Sports drinks are important to include in hydration plans for athletes who sweat heavily and for those who exercise in hot and humid conditions.

attention to what happens when their sweat dries after a workout. If you have ever noticed a gritty white residue left on your skin before showering or white streaks on your clothing, this is quite literally salt that was lost through sweat and has now dried. Although this is normal, salty sweaters tend to notice this more than the average athlete.

If you are a heavy or salty sweater, you should be purposeful about including electrolytes in your hydration and fueling plan. A common source of electrolytes around activity are sports drinks, which can be a great way to help replace both fluid and electrolytes at the same time. Look for a sports drink that has more sodium than any other electrolyte listed on the label. There are many electrolyte products in powder or liquid concentrate form that can be added to fluids. Keep in mind that many of these products bear a Supplements Facts label rather than a Nutrition Facts label; caution about these products will be discussed in chapter 8.

A few recommended products are listed in table 7.1, although these are far from the only ones available. Generally, the heavier of a sweater you are, the higher sodium content you should choose. Remember that carbohydrate content varies in sports drinks, especially depending on the brand. Make sure to choose a higher carbohydrate option when doing longer, more intense workouts, and lower carbohydrate options when doing lighter training. In addition to choosing a sodium level that fits your level of sweating, you should also choose a product that makes the most sense for the logistics of your workout (is a powdered packet easier to pack? A liquid packet or premixed bottle more convenient to use during a workout?). You may also need to try a few to determine your taste preferences.

When it comes to supplementing electrolytes, the products discussed in table 7.1 are great options, but of course come with a price. A much cheaper option can be to simply salt your food more at meals and snacks,

TABLE 7.1   **Electrolyte Levels in Fluid-Replacement Products**

Product	Sodium	Potassium
Gatorade (20 fl oz)	306 mg	135 mg
Powerade (12 fl oz)	240 mg	80 mg
Pedialyte Sport (12 fl oz)	490 mg	470 mg
Propel (20 fl oz)	270 mg	70 mg
Gatorlyte Rapid Rehydration (20 fl oz)	490 mg	350 mg
The Right Stuff (1 packet)	1,780 mg	0 mg
Liquid IV (1 packet)	500 mg	370 mg
DripDrop (1 packet)	330 mg	185 mg

especially if you are in a high training period or in a hot or humid environment for training. For more on sodium and electrolyte supplementation, see chapter 6.

Muscle Cramps

One of the more well known—and most uncomfortable—symptoms caused by dehydration is muscle cramps. Historically, athletes struggling with muscle cramps have been told to drink more fluids and replenish electrolytes to help prevent this unpleasant side effect, but more has been learned about the causes of cramping in recent years and the different approaches you may take depending on what's causing them.

Some muscle cramping is caused simply by overuse or fatigue of specific muscle groups, and not much can be done to prevent this other than using a stepwise approach with increased activity and a well-rounded strength and conditioning plan. This type of cramping is commonly seen early in the season or during preseason training when athletes come back after time off. This cramping is also commonly seen in muscle groups that are being heavily taxed, such as calf cramping when doing a lot of conditioning that requires repeated quick firing of the calf muscle, or perhaps arm or hand cramping for repetitive motions like pitching or throwing. Although it certainly won't hurt to hydrate well and include some electrolytes if you expect to sweat during the activity, these sorts of cramps can be unavoidable if the muscles are deconditioned.

Another common cause of cramping is inadequate fluid intake, which occurs when the decreased blood volume caused by dehydration results in decreased blood flow to muscles. As discussed previously, dehydration causes a whole host of issues with performance, but muscle cramping is certainly one that can motivate athletes to appropriately hydrate, because the consequences of not doing so are painful and immediate. From this standpoint, it's vital to get adequate fluid leading up to training or competitions. Urine should be light in color and you should not be notably thirsty. It's important to remember that drinking a bunch of water or other fluids right before competition or training does not adequately hydrate you—the body can only process fluid so quickly, and you will not actually absorb enough water to avoid problems.

In addition to inadequate fluid intake, inadequate electrolyte intake can also lead to muscular cramping. Because of the role electrolytes play in muscle contraction, the body's ability to send signals from the brain to the muscle can be interrupted when electrolytes are too low, causing the body to overcompensate by sending more signals. This can collectively result in the muscle becoming overstimulated and unable to relax as it normally would. Heavy sweaters should be especially purposeful about including electrolytes—notably sodium—around training and competition for this reason. Many heavy sweaters benefit from including at least 100 to 400 milligrams of sodium per hour, but rates are very individualized. Unfortunately, there is not a good way to quantify specific sodium needs without sweat testing, but many athletes can be successful through trial and error—another example of practicing your fueling plan during training so that you can perfect it for competition. By ensuring appropriate training progression and fluid and electrolyte intake, most athletes can avoid cramping completely. However, hydration approaches are preventative. Once you are already cramping, you should definitely consume fluid and electrolytes to help try to correct the imbalance, but these will not fix the problem very quickly for most athletes.

With all this in mind, some cramping is inevitable even with the most careful planning—perhaps you end up playing more minutes than usual or the weather is unusually hot or humid. Luckily, more recent research has provided insight on what can help once you're already cramping. Research conducted by Schwellnus (2009) suggests that exercise-associated muscle cramps (EAMCs) occur when fatigue and other risk factors contribute to an imbalance between excitatory and inhibitory stimuli at the motor nerve. I often describe this to athletes as a misfire between synapses in the brain and the muscles, which can lead to overexcitation of the nerves that cause muscle contraction. A review by Miller and colleagues (2022) notes that certain compounds like acetic acid and capsaicin can act on receptors in the mouth and esophagus and essentially "reset" this misfire. Foods with these compounds include pickle juice, apple cider, white vinegar, and products that include hot pepper juice or extract. The suggested use of these products is to swish a small amount of the fluid around your mouth for 15 to 20 seconds, then swallow it. You should only use these compounds when actively cramping and in small amounts as needed. Although it's difficult to tell what caused a cramp in hindsight, the best course of action is to take a preventative approach with adequate hydration, and in the (hopefully rare) instance where you still have cramping, you can take appropriate action.

Environment

There are many things that you can control in terms of hydration, but it's important to be aware of the things you cannot control—namely, the weather and environment. Although you can't control these things, you can at least prepare for them. Some of the most common environmental challenges and hydration strategies are discussed next.

Hot and Humid Temperatures

Because excess heat and humidity can contribute to substantially more fluid loss, you should prepare to sweat more and be ready to replace fluids appropriately in hot and humid conditions. A way to collectively measure heat and humidity is the heat index, and most athletes find that as heat index rises, so does their sweat rate. You should try to drink fluids every 15 to 20 minutes if possible and consider taking gulps instead of sips. You should also consider prioritizing sports drinks that contain electrolytes, which are likely to be lost at higher levels via the increased sweating. It can also be helpful to keep drinks cold with ice, which not only may make them more appealing but can also help keep your core temperature lower. This is important to help avoid heat stroke, a serious condition that can be fatal.

You have likely seen athletes dump water on themselves to cool off or perhaps have done this yourself. Although it might seem dramatic to some, this is actually an effective way to help your body stay cool. If training or competing in an extremely hot or humid environment you could consider bringing iced-down towels or cold water (separate from the water you plan to drink) for the purpose of cooling off. Dumping, splashing, or using cold wet towels on your head, neck, and torso areas can help keep core temperature down. If you ever feel like you are overheating and cannot get your temperature down, your heart races, or you become light-headed or dizzy, seek medical treatment immediately.

Cold Temperatures

Extremely cold temperatures can pose their own set of hydration problems. Although sweat rate tends to be significantly lower in colder weather, many athletes underestimate their hydration needs in cold weather. This can happen for a few different reasons. For one, thirst sensation is often lowered in cold weather, so athletes may not keep up with their needs simply because they don't feel thirsty. Another reason for underestimating fluid needs in the cold is because athletes often bundle up to help stay warm, which can lead to sweating more than they anticipate under all the layers. Finally, more water is lost through respiration in cold weather than in warmer weather. Picture "seeing your breath" when you walk outside in cold air—that is fluid leaving the body via respiration. Although this effect tends to be minimal, it can add up over a long period of activity or in conjunction with the other considerations mentioned. Try to stick to your normal hydration routine when exercising in colder weather, even if it doesn't seem like you need to.

Exercise in Water

Any swimmers reading may have already had the thought: "How am I supposed to assess my sweat rate when I'm always soaking wet?" This is a definite challenge for athletes in water sports. Many aspects of hydrating for these sports is no different than any other—you should try to hydrate consistently all day long and use urine color to assess hydration status leading up to and after activity. However, if you participate in a water sport and feel like you're struggling to appropriately hydrate or are experiencing symptoms associated with dehydration, it would be a good idea for you to use sweat rate testing methods described previously, such as taking a preworkout and postworkout weight (just ensure that you shower just before the preworkout weight so that it mimics what you'll be experiencing when you get out of the water). This will allow you to quantify your individual sweat loss per hour and make a plan to keep up with your fluid intake.

Altitude

The last example of an environmental situation that would potentially alter your hydration plan is training or competing at altitude (generally considered to be at or above 1,500 meters). Because respiration and urine fluid losses are increased at altitude (Saunders et al. 2019), total fluid intake should increase when training or competing at altitude. Although not related to hydration specifically, it should also be noted that total macronutrient and calorie needs are higher at altitude as a result of increased metabolic rate. Garvican-Lewis and colleagues (2016) also note that iron supplementation appears to be necessary for optimal adaptation to altitude—If you consistently train at altitude you should get your iron tested and supplement as indicated. If you don't regularly train at altitude but plan to compete at altitude you should consider supplementing iron in the weeks leading up to the competition. For specifics on iron supplementation, see chapter 6.

Hopefully you now have a better understanding of your hydration needs and how they can be individualized based on your preferences and your unique circumstances. Although some aspects of your hydration needs remain fairly consistent (body size, sex, propensity to sweat), other aspects may ebb and flow (weather, location, uniform). Be consistent with your approach, but be ready to pivot as needed and increase your fluid or electrolyte intake for that noon kickoff in the summer heat and humidity!

CHAPTER 8

Gain the Edge With Supplements

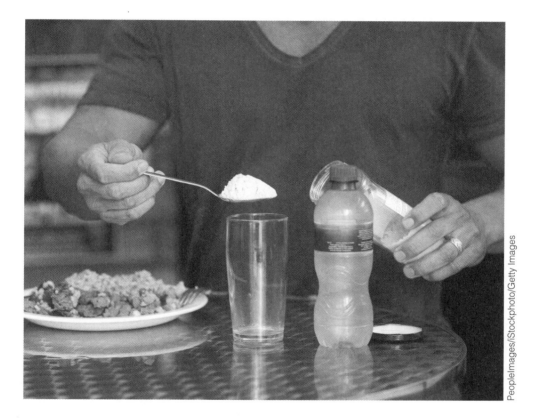

PeopleImages/iStockphoto/Getty Images

The world of dietary supplements is ever growing and ever changing. But before discussing whether you need supplements or what kinds of supplements might be right for your situation, it's important to understand what a supplement is. A dietary supplement is defined as a manufactured product intended to supplement a person's diet and is considered different from conventional food. Supplements span many different groups of nutrients. They may contain macronutrients, micronutrients, herbal ingredients, and everything in between.

Although some research indicates that athletes may have higher micronutrient needs than nonathletes as a result of high energy expenditure, physical stress, and loss of micronutrients via sweat, much of this research is not conclusive. Furthermore, as long as an athlete is eating enough food and their diet is relatively balanced, their higher caloric intake tends to provide higher micronutrient intake as well. However, as mentioned in chapter 6, these higher micronutrient needs along with limited diets and busy travel schedules mean that most athletes could probably benefit from a multivitamin supplement—as long as it's one that has undergone third-party testing (discussed next). This tends to be a safe approach to fill in any nutrient gaps that might exist in your diet.

Making Sense of Product Labeling

In the United States, an easy way to differentiate a supplement from a food or medicine is by checking the label on the back of the product. A supplement will have a Supplement Facts label, whereas a food will have a Nutrition Facts label and a medication will have a Drug Facts label. The critical difference between these three labels is that unlike food and medications, supplements are very poorly regulated by the U.S. Food and Drug Administration (FDA). In fact, there is essentially no premarket regulation of Supplement Facts labels, meaning that no one is required to check the safety, efficacy, or accuracy of these products before they are put on shelves. It would take a significant problem (and reporting of said problem) for a supplement to receive action from the FDA—generally speaking, it would take multiple people getting very sick or even dying. Even in the event of an issue, there is often very little follow-up or follow-through to ensure that appropriate changes have been made to the product before rolling it out again.

To put it plainly, if a product has a Supplement Facts label this means that the consumer cannot be sure the claims about the product are true nor that the ingredients listed are accurate or even safe. There may be more or less of the ingredients than are listed on the label, and there may even be something in the product that is not on the label at all. This is naturally concerning for health and safety reasons, but for athletes who are being drug tested by their program or its governing body, contamination from banned substances is a particular concern. If you're thinking the risk still seems pretty low, take note—one study by Crawford and colleagues (2022) analyzed 30 dietary supplements and found 17 of 30 had inaccurate labels: 13 were mislabeled, and 9 had additional components detected but not claimed on the label. This study is one of many with similar findings. These inaccuracies may be blatant and done with an intent of making a product work without disclosing the reason why the product is really working, or it may be caused by contamination from another company's product (it is extremely common for small companies to rent production facilities rather than having their own). You can also look for certain wording on supplement packaging or labels that indicate you should avoid the product—these red flags are listed in table 8.1.

TABLE 8.1   Red Flags to Look for on Supplement Labels

Label information	Red flag
Claims that sound too good to be true (e.g., "lose 10 pounds in 1 week!")	If it sounds too good to be true, it probably is.
Words like *proprietary* or *blend*	These allow companies to not disclose what exactly is in the blend or how much of each individual ingredient the blend contains.
Herbal ingredients	These are often thought of as safe because they're natural and come from plants. However, this is not necessarily the case, and many herbal ingredients (extracts, leaves, bark, roots, etc.) are very poorly regulated in their production and can have negative interactions with common medications, disease states, and even other herbal ingredients.
Claims around testosterone, estrogen, other hormones	Claims such as "testosterone boosting," "hormone altering," "the next best thing to steroids," or "barely legal" indicate the likely presence of dangerous (and often organizationally banned) ingredients.

Even purchasing a product from a reputable store does not give the product instant credibility. Regardless of where you bought it, the presence of a Supplement Facts label should make you pause and take some additional steps to ensure that the product is safe and necessary.

Luckily there are independent companies whose role is to test products against some of these concerns. The exact testing done depends on which third-party organization is doing the testing; some test for banned substances but not for accuracy of labeling, and vice versa. NSF International (formerly the National Sanitation Foundation) is one of the most well recognized of these organizations, and the NSF Certified for Sport certification (often referred to as the *gold standard*) confirms that the product has not only been proven to be free of banned substances, but that the label accurately reflects what is in the product. This is ideal for athletes, who should be concerned about banned substances in addition to general safety. It's important to look for labels specifically; some companies are notoriously sneaky and will make their own similar-looking versions of these labels with wording like "banned substance free," but these mean nothing.

Now that you know what a supplement is and what to look for, let's talk about whether you need one. It's important to remember that just because you have determined that a supplement is a quality product does not automatically mean that you should be using it. There are lots of things to consider when deciding if a supplement might be right for you. Some of these considerations are noted in table 8.2.

As the table suggests, any supplement you use should have third-party certification and should match your goals for using it. With this

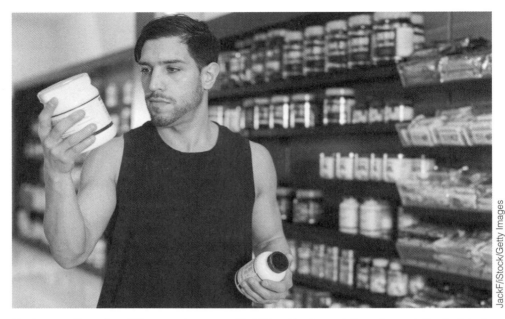

JackF/iStock/Getty Images

Understanding the difference between Nutrition Facts and Supplement Facts labels and the importance of third-party testing is vital for ensuring that products consumed are safe, legal, and efficacious.

TABLE 8.2   Questions to Consider Before Using Supplements

Consideration	Questions to ask yourself
Safety	Has it undergone third-party testing?
Dose	Is it an efficacious dose (enough to work but not enough to be dangerous)?
Ingredients	Is the form of the nutrient bioavailable or easily absorbed?
	Are there any ingredients that might inhibit absorption?
	Were the ingredients sourced in reputable conditions?
Cost	Is there a cheaper or equally effective way to get this nutrient?
Practicality	Does this supplement fit with my lifestyle and preferences?
	How and when will I use it, and is that realistic with my lifestyle and schedule?
Sport or training demands	Do the supplement's benefits or effects align with the demands of my training or sport?
	Does it support my body composition goals?

knowledge in hand, the rest of the chapter will discuss some of the most common supplements as well as considerations for their use and timing that can help maximize their effectiveness. Remember that vitamins and minerals were covered specifically in chapter 6.

Creatine

Creatine is a compound that supplies muscles with immediate energy for quick bursts of explosive movement. Your body produces some creatine (about 1 g/day), and animal products like meat and fish have naturally occurring creatine as well. Many athletes are interested in supplementing creatine, though, and for good reason. Supplemental creatine has been shown to increase the amount of creatine stored in muscle, which can lead to improvements in strength and power and improve overall maximal effort (Kreider et al. 2017). It's important to note that not everybody responds the same way to creatine. About one-third of people are considered nonresponders because they already have naturally high levels of creatine. The only way to know if you respond to supplemental creatine is to try it and see if you notice effects.

Research shows that taking creatine over several weeks or months is safe for adults (Antonio et al. 2021). There has historically been a gap in the research on the effect of long-term creatine use over many years, but as data continue to emerge it appears that long-term use is likely safe as well, with some researchers even referring to creatine as a life cycle supplement based on the idea that it can provide benefits across a person's entire life. The International Society of Sports Nutrition Position Stand also affirms the safety of creatine, citing long-term studies that show it is not harmful to organs (Kreider et al. 2017).

It is well known that creatine can improve performance during short intermittent bouts of intense activity (30-120 sec). Examples of movements that might be improved by use of creatine include sprinting, jumping, lifting, and throwing. Although creatine has never been considered to be very applicable to endurance activities like distance running, swimming, rowing, or cycling, emerging research has created interest in regard to creatine's effects on endurance performance as well. In fact, creatine supplementation can enhance glycogen supercompensation (Nelson et al. 2001), which could be an effective strategy for endurance athletes looking to maximize their carbohydrate-loading approach (detailed more in chapter 3).

Dosing

In terms of dosing creatine, you will often hear the terms *loading phase* and *maintenance phase*. The loading phase is used as a mechanism to build up creatine concentrations in the tissues and is often recommended at 20 grams per day for four to five days. For a more individualized dosing protocol, consuming 0.3 grams per kilogram for five days is effective for loading. After completing the loading phase it is recommended to transition to a lower dose in the maintenance phase—usually 3 to 5 grams per day. If you don't like the idea of consuming 20 grams of creatine per day, that's OK. If you consume the recommended maintenance dose, you will eventually build up tissue concentrations after about a month of supplementation. In a review of the literature, Antonio and colleagues (2021) mention specifically that smaller daily dosages of creatine supplementation (3-5 g or 0.1 g/kg of body mass) are effective.

There are a number of forms of creatine available on the market. However, creatine monohydrate is the most widely used and studied form of creatine in supplements; I recommend looking for one that is 100 percent creatine monohydrate. Creatine monohydrate is sometimes thought to not dissolve as well as other forms, but this slight inconvenience is well worth the superior efficacy of the form. If you struggle to get creatine to dissolve well in liquid, you can try using slightly warmer water or even mix it into yogurt or a smoothie.

Risk Factors

It is a common misconception that creatine causes muscle cramping and that you need to take extra care to hydrate well if you are using creatine. Although you should always try to ensure good hydration habits, the link between creatine and cramping specifically has been disproven. With any supplement, there is always potential for individual reactions like GI distress, but this is not a concern for most. If you experience these symptoms you should discontinue use. Because it is processed by the kidneys, you should talk to your doctor before using creatine if you suffer from kidney disease or only have one kidney.

Creatine for Women?

Many women are turned off by the idea of using creatine because they are fearful of weight gain and the idea of getting "bulky." Some also may have felt that they didn't experience performance effects from creatine supplementation. However, females often have higher concentrations of creatine in their muscles, possibly as a result of lower overall skeletal muscle mass, which may explain the lack of performance effects as compared to males. Females have also been reported to have lower levels of creatine in the brain (specifically the frontal lobe). By supplementing creatine and increasing this concentration, it may help reduce symptoms of depression and reduce severity of the effects of traumatic brain injury. Overall, research thoroughly supports women using creatine to support performance and health (Antonio et al. 2021).

One side effect you may notice is some water retention. It is this quick weight gain that sometimes gets athletes' attention and makes them think it is working. However, that acute weight gain caused by retained water does not reflect a change in performance—yet. It is through continued use and the ability to train harder and with more explosive movements that athletes see a long-term gain in muscle mass and ultimately performance.

In addition to performance and body composition, more recent literature has shown creatine's positive effect on many aspects of mental health and performance. Research by Machek and Bagley (2018) as well as Forbes and colleagues (2022) discusses positive impacts on cognitive parameters such as memory, focus, and attention. Research has also begun to establish that creatine may be neuroprotective if being taken consistently leading up to a brain injury (Dolan 2019). These findings have those who work in concussion-prone sports very excited about the potential to help attenuate some of the symptoms of concussion, as well as reduce the severity of a concussion and potentially reduce the number of days to recovery.

Timing

Although it is not uncommon to hear suggestions that creatine is most beneficial if taken before or after exercise, there is currently a lack of research showing that the timing of creatine ingestion has an impact on results (Candow et al. 2022). The most important factor for maximizing creatine's effects is to take it consistently and maintain the appropriate dosing. As mentioned previously, though there may be a small shift in water weight when you start taking creatine, the real benefits come from taking it consistently over time to build up the levels in your muscle tissue.

Collagen

Collagen peptides are short chains of amino acids derived from collagen, which is the most abundant form of structural protein in the body, found in tendons, ligaments, skin, and bones. Although the claims about the benefits of collagen span from hair, skin, and nail growth to soft-tissue injury management and everything in between, the current literature on the matter is less convincing. However, many practitioners do feel as though collagen can play a role in soft-tissue injury treatment and management for athletes. Collagen is often discussed in tandem with vitamin C because vitamin C is essential in the enzymatic reaction that converts individual amino acids proline and lysine into collagen fibers. Many collagen supplements come with vitamin C already added, but if you're using one that does not, then you should consider taking it with a vitamin C supplement or mixing it with fruit juice that is naturally high in vitamin C.

There are many different types of collagen in the body, but some of the most common are listed here. Dietary supplements often contain primarily type I collagen due to its abundance in the body, but the specific formulation used may depend on the brand and the product.

1. *Type I*. This is the most abundant type of collagen in the body, constituting around 90 percent of total collagen. It is found in the skin, bones, tendons, ligaments, and other connective tissues. Type I collagen provides strength, structural support, and flexibility to these tissues.

2. *Type II*. This type of collagen is primarily present in cartilage, which is the flexible connective tissue found in joints. Type II collagen contributes to the structural integrity and resilience of cartilage, providing cushioning and shock absorption.

3. *Type III*. Type III collagen is often found alongside type I collagen, providing structural support to organs, blood vessels, and tissues such as the skin and muscles. It plays a role in tissue repair and regeneration.

4. *Type IV*. Unlike the fibrillar collagens (types I, II, and III), type IV collagen forms a meshlike structure and is a major component of the basement membrane, which acts as a barrier and provides support to various tissues and organs, including the skin, blood vessels, and kidneys.

5. *Type V collagen*. Type V collagen is often found in association with type I collagen in tissues such as the skin, tendons, and ligaments. It helps regulate the assembly and organization of collagen fibers and contributes to the overall structure and stability of these tissues.

Dosing

A study by Clark and colleagues (2008) showed that administering 10 grams of collagen hydrolysate per day could help reduce the symptoms of joint pain associated with athletic activity as well as improve joint functionality. Another study by Lugo and colleagues (2013) showed that collagen supplementation increased the amount of time that the athletes were free of joint pain. A 5 to 15 grams per day dose of collagen taken at least one hour prior to exercise for at least three months could aid in reducing joint pain and improving muscle recovery—which could be integral in recovery from a soft-tissue injury. Given that supplemental collagen is most beneficial after consistent use for three months or more, athlete compliance to a supplementation plan is key.

Risk Factors

Although the research remains somewhat inconsistent, a third-party tested collagen supplement should be low risk and—if nothing else—an additional source of protein. In fact, for those who feel like collagen really improves their hair, skin, and nail growth, it's possible that it's simply the result of additional protein in their diet, especially if their diet lacked total protein or a variety of protein sources before the addition of collagen.

Timing

The research on timing of collagen specifically remains relatively limited. Similar to muscle protein synthesis (MPS) discussed in early chapters, collagen synthesis is a continuous process that occurs in the body over the course of an entire day. With this in mind, consistency in taking collagen supplements, rather than specific timing, is likely more important for achieving the benefits desired. However, there are some studies that have examined collagen supplementation specifically before exercise, including one by Shaw and colleagues (2017) that showed consuming a vitamin C–enriched gelatin supplement increased the serum amount of collagen-forming amino acids. Additionally, the subjects who consumed the gelatin one hour before rope-skipping for six minutes showed twice as much collagen synthesis as the placebo and low-gelatin groups.

Overall, the practicality of when athletes are able to realistically consume a collagen supplement and remember to do so consistently over a span of months should be the biggest factor influencing timing. However, if athletes are rehabbing a soft-tissue injury or taking a collagen supplement with the goal of supporting muscle growth, it may be advantageous to take it prior to a workout or rehabilitation session.

Caffeine

Caffeine is a stimulant that is commonly enjoyed through naturally derived sources like coffee and tea as well as through artificially caffeinated substances like energy drinks and supplements like preworkout powders. Caffeine can be ergogenic for performance if used appropriately, and its natural sources also have antioxidant properties. However, like many things, excessive caffeine can quickly become concerning and even dangerous. On the low end of risk, caffeine can cause dependance and corresponding withdrawal symptoms in some people. On the high end, caffeine can cause increased heart rate and blood pressure and in extreme instances can even cause cardiac arrest.

Caffeine is permitted by most athletic governing bodies, although sometimes with stipulations. For instance, the National Collegiate Athletic Association (NCAA) bans caffeine in urine concentrations over 15 micrograms per milliliter during competition. It takes 500 to 800 milligrams of caffeine, or about 5 to 8 cups of coffee consumed two to three hours before competition, for most people to achieve this urine concentration. Although extreme, it's important to remember that because people metabolize caffeine differently, the same amount may affect two people totally differently.

Dosing

Caffeine is considered "likely safe" by Natural Medicines Database when used orally and appropriately (Therapeutic Research Center 2023). Generally speaking, amounts up to 400 milligrams daily, or about 4 cups of coffee, are considered safe. For those who are pregnant or lactating this amount is lower, usually referenced around 200 milligrams, but you should always talk to your doctor for personal recommendations. When evaluating a food product's label, it's important to remember that only the amount of added caffeine has to be listed. If the food naturally contains caffeine. that amount does not have to be listed (though it often is), making it potentially difficult to determine the total amount of caffeine in a given product. It is also common to see caffeine listed as part of a proprietary blend, meaning you cannot be sure how much of the total blend is made up from caffeine.

Risk Factors

Caffeine is considered to be "possibly unsafe" when used long term or in high doses. Acute use of doses above 400 milligrams per day has been associated with adverse health effects like increased heart rate, heart palpitations, and sleep disturbances. Caffeine is considered to be "likely unsafe" when used in very high doses. A dose of 10 to 14 grams (10,000-14,000 mg) is considered to be a fatal dose, but serious toxicity can occur at lower doses, especially depending on the individual (Therapeutic Research Center 2023).

Timing

It is important to approach caffeine with moderation and monitor your personal reaction to it. However, it must be acknowledged that caffeine's effects span past just helping you stay awake; research has thoroughly

Energy Drinks and Caffeine

As mentioned above, one common method of caffeine delivery is via energy drinks. Energy drinks tend to toe the line on FDA regulation, in that some have a Nutrition Facts label while others have a Supplement Facts label. Regardless of what type of label they use, many energy drinks contain ingredients that are important to be aware of if you are someone who enjoys them. I recommend that you look for a third-party label on energy drinks just as you would a supplement. This certification can help you feel confident not only about the ingredients, but also that the amount of caffeine being touted on the label matches what is found in the product. Table 8.3 breaks down some other common ingredients found in energy drinks and some important considerations around them.

TABLE 8.3   COMMON INGREDIENTS IN ENERGY DRINKS

Ingredient	Potential Benefits	Concerns
Caffeine	Increased alertness and focus	Potential for addiction, increased heart rate and blood pressure, disrupted sleep patterns, dehydration
Taurine	Improved exercise performance, enhanced cognitive function	Limited research, potential interactions with medications, possible cardiovascular effects
Guarana extract	Increased energy and mental alertness	Similar concerns as caffeine (contains caffeine)
B vitamins	Enhanced energy metabolism, improved nervous system function	High doses may cause niacin flush, potential for interactions with medications
Ginseng	Improved cognitive function, increased energy	Possible interactions with medications, stimulant effects, potential for elevated blood pressure
Sugar and sweeteners	Quick source of energy, improved taste	High sugar content can contribute to weight gain, tooth decay; artificial sweeteners may have health concerns
Artificial flavoring	Enhanced taste and variety	Some artificial flavors may have potential health risks
Preservatives	Extended shelf life and product stability	Some preservatives may have potential health risks
Carbonation	Enhanced sensory experience	Can cause bloating, stomach discomfort, and dental erosion

shown that caffeine does have an ergogenic effect on performance. A review by Guest and colleagues (2021) highlights that caffeine can show small to moderate improvements in muscular endurance and strength; sprinting, jumping, and throwing performance; and a wide range of aerobic and anaerobic sport-specific actions. Aerobic endurance appears to have the largest positive performance effects. One study by Grgic and colleagues (2019) found that different doses of caffeine enhanced both upper and lower body strength and that all doses improved lower body muscle endurance. When looking for ergogenic effects from caffeine, it is recommended to consume 3 to 6 milligrams per kilogram of body weight about 60 minutes before beginning exercise.

If you are looking to supplement caffeine, starting with whole food is generally a safer and a more moderate approach. 1 cup (8 fl oz) of coffee has about 100 milligrams of caffeine, which is a good starting point if you have not used caffeine in the past. Tea has less—around 25 milligrams per cup—but could still elicit a response in some people. If you don't enjoy these beverages or need a supplemental form for the sake of convenience, I would recommend an energy drink or third-party approved supplement with a moderate amount of caffeine (100-200 mg). There is also research to support that caffeine gum can be effective; a study by Lane and colleagues (2014) showed that participants receiving the caffeine via chewing gum saw a 3.9 percent performance improvement. Van Cutsem and colleagues (2018) also found improvements in reaction time, cognitive control, and countering mental fatigue with the use of a caffeine mouth-rinse, although more study is needed in this area—they found no effect on cognitive performance and did not take any whole-body performance measures.

Whatever the method of caffeine delivery, it is important to stick to one at a time: Caffeine stacking, or using multiple caffeine-containing products in a short amount of time, can lead to negative health effects.

Omega-3 Fatty Acids

Although there are plenty of foods that are rich in omega-3 fatty acids (covered in chapter 5), they are also available in supplemental form. These are of particular interest to athletes because of their anti-inflammatory and neuroprotective properties, and because fatty fish and seafood—primary sources of omega-3 fatty acids—are not always easy to include in athletes' diets. Philpott and colleagues (2018) found that omega-3 supplementation may improve the markers of muscle damage and soreness in team sport athletes. Although athletes can benefit from omega-3 supplementation at any point (especially if their diet is not high in omega-3s), they can especially be of interest in helping to promote healing and manage inflammatory states when undergoing high training loads, putting stress on certain joints, or recovering from injury.

There is also emerging research to support the use of omega-3 supplements for protective care in athletes who are prone to concussions. Although supplements of course cannot prevent a concussion, consistently using omega-3s can help athletes reduce severity and symptoms if they do sustain a concussion. It is recommended to continue using omega-3s after sustaining a concussion to help treat the symptoms (Lewis 2016). In addition to third-party testing, you might also evaluate the ratio of eicosapentaenoic acid (EPA) to docosahexaenoic acid (DHA). If you are looking to manage inflammation, an ideal ratio is around 2-to-1. If your focus is on brain health or recovery from a concussion, research suggests that more DHA than EPA is likely beneficial.

Dosing

More research is needed to determine an optimal dose of omega-3s. Current research utilizes a wide range—most using anywhere from 1.8 to 3 grams per day of combined EPA and DHA. Although there is not a formal UL established for omega-3 fatty acids, generally 5 grams per day would be considered the maximum appropriate amount. More research is also needed regarding how long omega-3 fatty acids should be taken to see improvements, but Philpott, Witard, and Galloway (2019) suggest that at least two weeks is needed to see increased omega-3 in the muscle.

If your diet is low in omega-3s, you are in a high training period, or you play a sport that puts a lot of stress on your joints or makes you prone to concussion, it would be appropriate to consider taking an omega-3 fatty acid supplement that has undergone third-party testing. An appropriate dose would be between 1 and 3 grams per day, with a 2-to-1 EPA to DHA ratio. If you are managing a concussion, however, that ratio can be reversed. Ultimately, research regarding these ratios and the stipulations that surround them is still fairly new. If you are unsure which supplement best suits your needs, aim for one containing a balance of EPA and DHA and take the total recommended dose. Ideally you would take this consistently to keep levels up and help mitigate inflammation and prevent injury, not just after you sustain an injury.

Risk Factors

Although omega-3 supplementation is generally considered safe when taken in appropriate doses, there are a few considerations that are important to be aware of. The first is that omega-3 fatty acids (especially DHA and EPA) have mild blood-thinning properties. This can be a positive for overall cardiovascular health, but can increase the risk for bleeding. Individuals who are on blood thinners or who have bleeding disorders should consult with their physician. Similarly, if you're planning to have surgery you should make sure to disclose to your physician that you are taking omega-3 supplements regularly. It's possible they will want you to discontinue for one to two weeks leading up to surgery just to eliminate this small risk. In addition to blood thinners, omega-3 fatty acids can also interact with antiplatelet drugs and some cholesterol medications, potentially altering their efficacy or safety. As with the other examples, make sure to have a conversation with your physician.

Another group that should use caution when considering omega-3 supplements is anyone who has a seafood or shellfish allergy. Because fish and shellfish are common sources of omega-3 fatty acids, a better option for anyone with an allergy would be to use an omega-3 supplement sourced from algae.

Lastly, though not a risk, per se, it is important to note that a common side effect of omega-3 supplementation is the fishy taste (and sometimes fishy burps) that accompany it! Although this is totally normal, it can be very off-putting for some people. Keeping the fish oil in the refrigerator or freezer can help blunt the taste profile, and consuming with food can help keep the unpleasant taste at bay if this bothers you.

Timing

There are not currently any definitive guidelines around timing of omega-3 supplementation. Like many other examples, taking it consistently is far more important than the specific time it's taken. Some people find it to be more palatable with food, but otherwise timing should be based around when you are best able to consistently take the supplement.

Carbohydrate Supplements

The importance of carbohydrate has been discussed many times throughout this book, and certainly many athletes have plenty of carbohydrate-rich foods that work well for them and their training routine. However, there are many carbohydrate supplements on the market that can be extremely helpful for athletes looking to increase carbohydrate intake in an efficient and convenient manner. Like any fueling routine, you should try these products during training and see what works for you before using them in a competition.

Carbohydrate gels and chews are a convenient way to get in a significant amount (often 20-30 g) of simple carbohydrates quickly. These simple carbohydrates tend to be easily digested and easy on the stomach, making them perfect for just before or during training or competition. Remember that carbohydrates are broken down into simple sugars, some of which are transferred into the bloodstream to be delivered to the muscles for energy. This rise in blood glucose is then followed by insulin being released into the bloodstream, which functions to remove any excess glucose from the blood and store it as fat. Although these processes are sometimes viewed negatively, they are normal and not something that you need to fear if you are balancing your diet and eating based on your expenditure.

Carbohydrate powders are also popular and can function to add additional carbohydrate to pre- and postworkout routines for athletes with high energy expenditures. Some of these products are advertised as "modified carbohydrates" and contain starches, often cornstarch, that have been structurally modified to elicit a different response in the gut. These modified starches can provide more long-lasting energy because they are digested more slowly and therefore cause a muted blood glucose and insulin spike. If used consistently and appropriately this could promote a shift toward a leaner body composition because the fat-storing function of insulin is diminished. Although this can be appealing to some athletes, the overall effect is small and something I tend to only recommend to athletes who need a substantial amount of carbohydrate but are trying to make a shift in their body composition. Getting an appropriate amount of total carbohydrate will be more impactful to performance than using modified starches.

Dosing

There are a number of different considerations when it comes to dosing for carbohydrates, depending on the form and the situation. Refer to chapter 3 for carbohydrate-specific recommendations and chapters 10 and 11 for sport-specific recommendations. Any time you are consuming large amounts of carbohydrate, it's important to ensure that you are consuming adequate fluids as well. Carbohydrate (especially certain types of sugars like fructose) draw water into the gut, which can cause GI upset and contribute to dehydration leading up to or during activity. Specific recommendations for hydration can be found in chapter 7.

Risk Factors

Remember that if you are using a modified starch for the purpose of muted glucose effects, it's important to use by itself; consuming another carbohydrate with it would negate the effect that you are looking to elicit.

Some athletes find it to be easier on their stomach than other options, particularly when used 30 to 60 minutes prior to training. Because of the slower digestion rate, some athletes do not tolerate it well if consumed during training. Like most parts of a sports nutrition routine, you should trial your plan before game day to ensure that you don't experience GI distress.

Timing

Similar to dosing, many of the considerations for timing carbohydrate supplements have been spelled out in chapters 3, 10, and 11. But as a general rule, they should be used more heavily in the time frame leading up to competition or training and spaced out throughout the duration of the activity—especially if that activity will last more than two hours.

Protein Supplements

Although protein powders have been discussed briefly in other chapters, as one of the most commonly used supplements among athletes it's worth diving further into here. Similar to carbohydrate supplements, many foods in our diet provide ample protein. However, protein powders, shakes, and bars can provide a convenient and shelf-stable option for busy athletes on the go. Protein powders can also help add additional protein to foods you're already eating, which is especially helpful for athletes who eat no or limited meat. Not surprisingly, there are many kinds of protein supplements; the most common will be discussed here.

Types

Protein powders, shakes, and bars can vary between being classified as a supplement or a food, so it's important to give the label a look. If it has a Nutrition Facts label, you can feel confident about the safety of the product, though some products (especially powders) will still have a label for third-party testing, which is an added layer of security.

Whey

The most widely discussed protein supplement is whey protein, and for good reason. Whey protein is derived from milk and is considered a complete protein, meaning it has all the amino acids your body needs. It is especially well known for its high leucine content, an amino acid that is crucial in kickstarting the MPS process. You have probably noticed a few different types of whey protein product are available: whey protein concentrate, whey protein isolate, and whey protein hydrolysate. All of these are good options, but understanding the differences can help you make the right choice for your situation.

Whey protein concentrate can vary the most widely of the three in terms of protein content. Whey protein can be labeled as concentrate if 25 to 80 percent of its content by weight is protein. This wide variability usually lends itself to a cheaper price tag, but ultimately less protein by weight compared to its counterparts. On the other hand, whey protein isolate must have at least 90 percent of its weight come from protein, making it a purer, more protein-dense form. If you are really relying on the protein supplement to fill gaps in your diet, then I would recommend opting for an isolate product—especially if price is not a limiting factor. An isolate also tends to have less than 1 percent lactose, which makes it an ideal choice for athletes with lactose intolerance or sensitivities (though still not safe for those with a true dairy allergy). The last option is whey protein hydrolysate, which means it has been partially broken down and is therefore easier to digest. A hydrolysate product is absorbed more quickly than the others, but there is not a strong body of research to suggest that this makes it any better for MPS or recovery.

Casein

Another common protein supplement is casein. Similar to whey, casein is also derived from milk and is also considered a high-quality protein that contains all the amino acids. The primary difference between whey and casein is the rate at which they are absorbed. Casein is digested and therefore absorbed significantly more slowly. In a postworkout time frame when the goal is to efficiently promote recovery, this is not necessarily the best option. However, this slow absorption time makes casein an excellent choice for bedtime, because it slowly breaks down and releases amino acids into the bloodstream for four to five hours after digestion.

Plant-Based Protein

There are a number of different plant-based protein powders on the market, which are a good option for vegetarian or vegan athletes. It is recommended to use a pea or soy protein, which tend to be the most comparable to animal-based products in terms of protein and amino acid content.

Plant-based protein powders may also vary in their digestibility, which is important to be aware of. Some individuals may find plant-based protein powders harder to digest as a result of the fiber content and may experience bloating or other digestive symptoms. As with any product, trialing different options during training is recommended.

Dosing

When looking for a protein supplement, look for one that has 15 to 30 grams of protein per serving, makes sense for your lifestyle or logistical challenges, and either has a Nutrition Facts label or has undergone third-party testing.

Risk Factors

The primary risk factors associated with protein powders are those regarding the safety of supplements in general, as discussed at the beginning of the chapter. Protein powders have possibly a higher risk of being adulterated due to the fact that they often tout muscle growth and weight gain, and therefore may be more prone to companies using hormone-altering or other pharmaceutical ingredients to elicit such results.

Timing

As covered in chapter 4, the primary timing consideration for utilizing a protein powder or shake is taking advantage of the anabolic window within the first hour or two after a workout. However, one of the nice things about protein powders and shakes is their convenience—so not only are they great for the postworkout time frame, they can also help with the goal of eating protein consistently throughout the day, especially for busy athletes on the go.

Dietary Nitrates

Dietary nitrate is a compound found naturally in certain foods, such as leafy green vegetables, beetroot, and other root vegetables. When consumed, dietary nitrate is converted into nitric oxide, which plays a key role in various physiological processes. Notably, nitric oxide is a vasodilator, meaning it relaxes and widens blood vessels, leading to increased blood flow and oxygen delivery to the muscles. This can enhance exercise performance, particularly during endurance activities, by improving oxygen utilization, reducing the oxygen cost of exercise, and increasing exercise tolerance. In a review of 80 studies examining dietary nitrates' ability to improve aerobic performance, Senefeld and colleagues (2020) noted approximately 3 percent improvement in performance, though they did note that the studies predominantly included young men and that more research is needed on the topic for women specifically. Tan and colleagues (2022) also found that dietary nitrate supplementation may be effective in improving power and velocity in explosive resistance exercises (e.g., weightlifting) as well as the sprint time of explosive repeated sprint-type exercises (e.g., cycling and running), though continued research is needed in this area as well.

Dosing

The dosing of dietary nitrate can vary depending on the specific goals and preferences of the individual. Studies have shown that a daily intake of 6 to 8 millimoles (approximately 400-500 mg) of dietary nitrate, typically obtained from concentrated beetroot juice or nitrate-rich supplements, can produce beneficial effects on exercise performance (McMahon, Leveritt, and Pavey 2017). However, it is important to note that individual responses may vary, and it is advisable to experiment with different doses to determine your optimal amount.

Risk Factors

Dietary nitrate is generally considered safe for most individuals when consumed in moderate amounts, especially from natural food sources. However, it is important to note that excessive nitrate intake from supplements or certain processed foods may have potential health risks. Nitrate-rich foods should also be consumed as part of a balanced and varied diet to ensure optimal nutrient intake.

It can also be helpful to mention that consuming multiple servings of nitrate supplements like beet juice can also cause your urine to be red. So if you're supplementing with beet juice and notice this when you go to the bathroom, don't panic! This is a normal byproduct of your body breaking down the beets.

Timing

Timing of dietary nitrate consumption is also important. It has generally been recommended to consume nitrate-rich foods or supplements approximately two to three hours prior to exercise. This timing allows for peak nitric oxide levels to be reached during exercise, maximizing the potential performance benefits. More recent studies have shown that they may be beneficial even closer to activity, with some protocols evaluating dietary nitrate consumption 75 minutes prior to activity and showing positive results (Stecker et al. 2019).

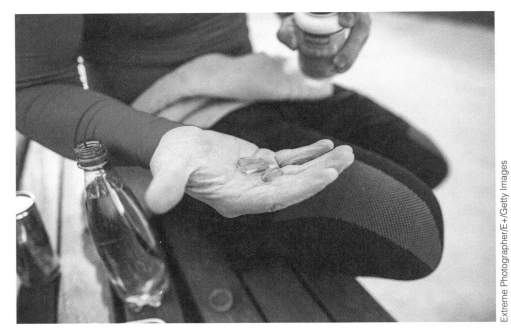

Extreme Photographer/E+/Getty Images

While supplements can help correct deficiencies and fill gaps in the diet, they should be viewed as a supplement to diet, not as a primary approach.

Beta-Alanine

Beta-alanine is a nonessential amino acid, meaning it can be synthesized by the body but can also be obtained through dietary sources and supplementation. Beta-alanine plays a role in the synthesis of carnosine, a protein molecule found in skeletal muscle that acts as a buffer to help regulate pH levels during intense exercise. By maintaining optimal pH levels, carnosine can help delay the onset of muscle fatigue and improve exercise capacity, particularly during short-duration, high-intensity activities.

Beta-alanine has consistently been shown to improve high-intensity exercise lasting between 1 and 10 minutes, lessen fatigue in both men and women, and increase resistance training volume. However, beta-alanine appears to work best in nontrained individuals—highly trained athletes may see less of an effect from using it.

Dosing

The dosing of beta-alanine sometimes involves a loading phase followed by a maintenance phase. During the loading phase, individuals consume around 4 to 6 grams of beta-alanine per day for a period of 4 to 6 weeks.

This loading phase helps to saturate the muscle stores of carnosine. Following the loading phase, a lower maintenance dose of around 2 to 3 grams per day is typically recommended to maintain the elevated carnosine levels. Saunders and colleagues (2017) point out that the research currently does not support that this loading protocol is really beneficial. They instead suggest that supplementation of 1.6 grams per day for as little as 2 weeks has been shown to increase muscle carnosine, while improvements in exercise have been shown at doses ranging from 3.2 to 6.4 grams per day for 4 to 12 weeks.

Risk Factors

Risk factors associated with beta-alanine are minimal. Some individuals may experience a tingling or flushing sensation known as *paresthesia* shortly after consuming beta-alanine. This sensation is harmless and temporary. Some individuals may also experience GI distress.

Timing

Timing of beta-alanine supplementation is not as critical as some other supplements, and there is currently not research available around timed delivery of beta-alanine to improve performance. As with many other examples, consistency is important to saturate levels in the muscle, so timing should be when you are best able to remember to take it. Because paresthesia, or flushing, is the most commonly reported side effect for athletes using beta-alanine (Stecker et al. 2019) and tends to occur when a large dose is taken at once (usually 800 mg or more), it can be beneficial to divide the total daily dose into smaller doses to help avoid the flushing. It can be taken at any time during the day, with or without food.

L-Citrulline

L-citrulline is an amino acid that is often used as a dietary supplement to potentially enhance exercise performance and promote overall cardiovascular health. It is often mentioned along with watermelon, because the fruit is naturally rich in it! It plays a crucial role in the urea cycle, which is a metabolic pathway involved in the removal of ammonia (a waste byproduct) from the body. It is also a precursor to another amino acid called L-arginine, which serves as a precursor for the production of nitric oxide. As discussed above, nitric oxide has a variety of important roles in the body, many of which can positively affect exercise performance. Currently the research regarding L-citrulline and strength exercise is small but growing. Evidence currently supports that citrulline doses over

3 grams result in small but statistically significant improvements for high-intensity strength and power performance (Gonzalez and Trexler 2020).

Dosing

The literature on L-citrulline recommends varying dosages, though typical dosages tend to be between 3 and 6 grams per day. Some studies have used higher dosages, upward of 8 to 15 grams per day, and appear to be well tolerated. Gonzalez and Trexler (2020) mention that based on the current evidence, chronic dosing over seven days seems to be more effective than an acute single-dose protocol for enhancing exercise performance. The minimum effective dose seems to be approximately 3 grams per day, whereas the maximum effective dose may be as high as 10 to 15 grams per day. Gonzalez and Trexler (2020) also mention that the combined effect of L-citrulline and L-arginine supplementation may have a more beneficial effect than a single dose of either amino acid alone.

Risk Factors

L-citrulline is generally considered safe for most people when taken in appropriate doses. It can interact with medications that lower blood pressure or treat erectile dysfunction, so you should consult with your health care provider before using an L-citrulline supplement if you are on these or similar medications.

Some people report GI distress when using L-citrulline supplements, so if you do experience those symptoms you should discontinue use. It's important to point out that GI distress is more common in people taking citrulline-malate supplements, which is a similar supplement but is not L-citrulline in its pure form.

Timing

Ingestion of L-citrulline 60 to 90 minutes before beginning exercise seems the best recommendation to reliably improve performance (Gonzalez and Trexler 2020). Future research should aim to examine the performance effects of both acute and chronic supplementation.

Nootropics

Nootropics are a relatively newer class of supplement that has gained momentum over the last 5 to 10 years. Sometimes referred to as *smart drugs*, they reference a diverse group of medicinal substances that have the potential to improve cognitive aspects of performance like focus, memory, critical thinking, and learning. The data suggest that these are much more effective in cases where baseline mental function is impaired in some way, but there remains a great deal of interest in the potential for healthy individuals to benefit as well (Schifano et al. 2022).

Nootropics function by improving the brain's supply of glucose and oxygen and protecting brain tissue from harmful effects. They may also positively affect the synthesis of phospholipids (certain types of lipid molecules needed for membranes in the brain). Some nootropics are synthetic, whereas many are of natural origin from various plants and herbs. Despite there being dozens of products that are purported to have nootropic properties, most still lack research to support their effects. In terms of synthetic compounds (e.g., Piracetam, Phenotropil, Noopept), they tend to have varying safety, especially when used over long periods of time, and many have been discontinued from commercial production. Additionally, though a few synthetic nootropic compounds show promise for things like anxiety, none currently have great evidence that they are effective in promoting athletic performance. This chapter will only discuss nootropics that are supported with sufficient data.

Types

When it comes to herbal compounds with purported nootropic effects, it's important to remember the discussion at the beginning of this chapter in terms of safety around supplements in general, herbals being no exception. Although there are some encouraging studies on the herbal nootropics highlighted here, most of them have not been studied in regard to long-term effects, and as such it may be advisable to only use for a limited time frame. Additionally, all of the following examples have interactions with at least one common medication such as blood pressure medications, blood thinners, ADHD medications, and many others. Finally, it is rare—though not impossible—to find herbal nootropics that have undergone third-party testing. If you are considering using an herbal supplement for its nootropic effects, you should look for a quality product with third-party testing, and if you are on any medication, discuss it with your doctor before starting.

Ginseng

Ginseng (also known as *panax ginseng*) is considered "likely safe" by Natural Medicines Database when used orally for up to six months (Therapeutic Research Center 2023). There is some concern around hormonelike effects when used long term. The exact mechanisms of how ginseng works are not fully understood, but it is thought to have adaptogenic properties, meaning it may help the body adapt to stressors and promote overall well-being. It may be effective for improving cognitive function, though most research shows that oral ginseng does not improve athletic performance.

Ginseng is typically used in doses of 200 milligrams to 3 grams daily for up to 12 weeks. Because ginseng is thought to have potential stimulant effects, there may be an amplified effect when combined with caffeinated food or drinks, such as coffee and tea. Until more research is done, it's advised to avoid taking ginseng with caffeine (ibid. 2023).

Ginkgo

Also known as *ginkgo biloba*, the leaf extract of ginkgo is considered "likely safe" when used orally and appropriately (the seeds and crude extract have some toxic constituents and should be avoided), and research supports its safe use for up to six years. Ginkgo is thought to enhance the flow of blood and oxygen to the brain, which may contribute to improved cognitive function, memory, and concentration. Ginkgo is also believed to have antioxidant properties, which can help protect cells from damage. It may also be effective for helping with anxiety and vertigo, but does not have any solid body of research to support improving athletic performance (ibid. 2023).

Ashwagandha

Ashwagandha is considered "possibly safe" when used orally and appropriately over the short term. Ashwagandha has been used in doses of up to 1,250 milligrams daily for up to six months without concerns for safety or adverse effects (ibid. 2023). It also has antioxidant properties, which can help protect the body's cells from damage. Ashwagandha may have neuroprotective properties and can support cognitive processes such as memory, attention, and information processing. It has also been shown to improve cognitive performance in tasks requiring attention and reaction time. Additionally, ashwagandha may be effective for helping improve insomnia and relieve stress and anxiety by reducing the levels of certain stress hormones like cortisol, which can indirectly enhance mental performance and focus. It is unclear if ashwagandha is beneficial for improving athletic performance, though more recent research has piqued interest due to potential positive implications for performance.

A meta-analysis of four small clinical trials by Pérez-Gómez and colleagues (2020) showed that taking ashwagandha increased aerobic capacity in athletes, based on the measurement of maximum oxygen consumption. Doses ranged from 500 to 1,000 milligrams daily for up to 12 weeks. A different meta-analysis by Bonilla et al. (2021) showed that doses of 120 to 1,250 milligrams as either a single dose or in two doses daily for up to six months appeared to improve muscle strength, speed, time to exhaustion, recovery time, and aerobic fitness in athletes. However, researchers agree that more studies are needed with better constraints around control groups and the wide variance in doses used, fitness level of participants, and outcomes assessed.

Rhodiola

Rhodiola is considered "possibly safe" when used orally and appropriately over the short term. Dosages that appear in research are up to 300 to 600 milligrams for up to 12 weeks without adverse effects (Therapeutic Research Center 2023). Rhodiola is believed to regulate levels of certain neurotransmitters in the brain, including serotonin, dopamine, and norepinephrine, which are involved in regulating mood, attention, and other cognitive processes. By influencing these neurotransmitters, rhodiola may improve mental alertness, focus, and concentration. Rhodiola is also believed to have neuroprotective effects, meaning it may help protect brain cells from damage caused by oxidative stress and inflammation.

The research to support rhodiola's positive effects on athletic performance is limited, but there are a few studies that indicate promising effects on certain aspects of performance. One by De Bock and colleagues (2004) indicates that 200 milligrams of rhodiola before exercise can improve endurance exercise capacity. In general, it appears that acute doses of rhodiola may improve specific physical performance parameters like time to exhaustion, peak oxygen use, time to completion, perceived exhaustion, anaerobic capacity, and power, although neither acute nor chronic doses appear to notably improve muscle function.

Phosphatidylcholine

A group of supplements related to nootropics is cholinergics, which help form acetylcholine, an important cofactor in processes related to many different cognitive functions. The primary cholinergic discussed is phosphatidylcholine, a type of phospholipid, which are crucial components of cell membranes.

Phosphatidylcholine is a major component of lecithin, which is found in foods like soybean and sunflower oil, as well as egg yolks, liver, whole grains, and some nuts. Phosphatidylcholine has been shown to quickly replenish choline levels or even negate depletion if supplemented prior to exercise (Jäger, Purpura, and Kingsley 2007). This is of interest to researchers because exercise lowers choline levels, which could affect endurance and overall performance. Supplementally, phosphatidylcholine is considered "possibly safe" when used orally and appropriately.

With that said, the research remains inconclusive as to whether true performance benefits are seen from phosphatidylcholine supplementation.

However, is it generally agreed that with the increasing popularity of low-fat diets, it's possible that many athletes don't get as many phospholipids from their diet as they once may have and may especially benefit from use of supplemental phosphatidylcholine.

Dosing

Dosing for nootropics is dependent on each individual substance and should be approached individually. Because many of these ingredients still lack a solid body of evidence, you should only take supplements that have undergone third-party testing, start with the lowest effective dose, and gradually increase only if needed. As with any new supplement, you should discuss with a dietitian or health care provider prior to taking—especially if you are on any kind of medication or have underlying conditions.

Risk Factors

With a category of supplements that represents a wide range of different products and ingredients, it is not surprising that the risk factors for nootropics depend a fair amount on the ingredient itself. However, as a general summary, some risk factors associated with nootropics include increased blood pressure and heart rate, sleep disturbances, trouble with vision, and sometimes GI distress. You should always consult your physician on anything else you're taking—especially when considering prescription nootropics— to know whether it may or may not be appropriate for you.

Timing

Timing with nootropics depends on the individual supplement and the purpose for which you are taking it. Some people may choose to take nootropics in the morning to enhance focus and mental clarity throughout the day. Others may prefer to take them in the afternoon to combat afternoon fatigue or support cognitive performance during demanding tasks. It's generally recommended to follow the instructions provided with the specific nootropic supplement or consult with a health care professional for personalized guidance.

Although supplements can potentially enhance athletic performance, it is important for athletes to exercise caution and always make informed decisions when considering supplements. Several key points should be considered to ensure the safe and effective use of supplements.

First, athletes should prioritize a well-balanced and nutrient-dense diet as the foundation of their nutritional strategy. Supplements should be viewed as complements to rather than substitutes for a healthy diet. Second, athletes should be cautious when selecting and using supplements, ensuring they come from reputable sources and are third-party tested. It is important to carefully read and understand product labels; consider individual needs, goals, and specific dietary restrictions; and consult with a registered dietitian, if possible.

Finally, athletes should be aware of the potential risks and limitations associated with supplement use. Not all supplements have solid scientific evidence to support their claimed benefits, and some may even carry potential health risks or contraindications. It's important to rely on evidence-based research and be critical of marketing claims when considering a new supplement.

Now that you have all of the pieces of the performance puzzle, it's time to make them fit together around your training!

PART II

Fine-Tune Your Fueling for Any Schedule

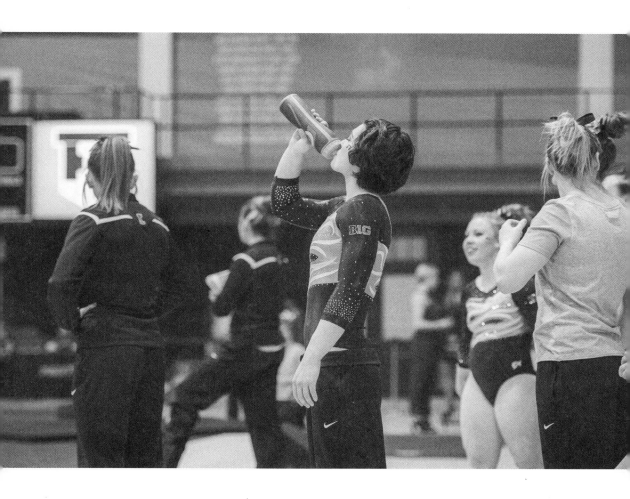

CHAPTER 9
Strategies for Training and Competition

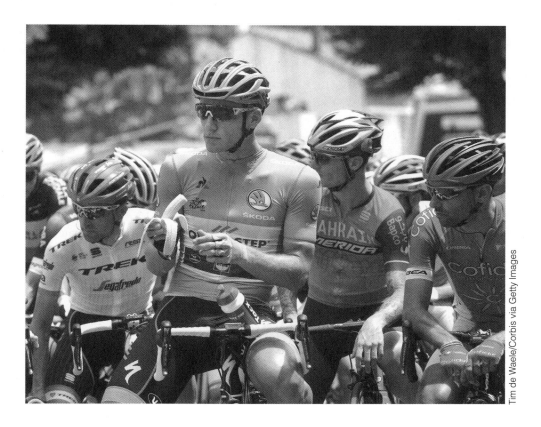

Tim de Waele/Corbis via Getty Images

Nutrient timing is crucial for many aspects of athletic success, but perhaps none more so than the time frames leading up to, during, and immediately after training and competition. Appropriate nutrient timing can not only ensure that you have the right kind and right amount of fuel on board, but also that you minimize GI discomfort that can interfere with optimal performance. Over time, appropriate nutrient timing around training also helps promote a lean body composition by supporting MPS. This chapter will discuss the specific elements of each time frame surrounding the workout.

Preworkout Nutrition

Preworkout nutrition has been covered briefly in other chapters, but a proper preworkout fueling routine is worth discussing in detail! I often describe this time frame to athletes like a funnel. At the top of the funnel is three to four hours before the workout or competition. At this point, this meal should look like the balanced plate discussed all the way back in chapter 2, with a balance of carbohydrate, lean protein, and fruit or veggies plus water or another hydrating fluid. Although this meal can be a little more relaxed than something being consumed closer to training or competition, you should generally choose foods that you know your stomach handles well—especially if this meal is happening on a competition day. Game day is not the time to try new foods. Instead, use training days to trial your fueling plan and ensure that certain foods work well for you. It is also generally advisable to avoid spicy foods and keep choices fairly lean (avoid fried foods, creamy or cheesy sauce, and high-fat meats like ribs, bacon, sausage, or wings). As mentioned in chapter 3, if you're three to four hours out from activity you should aim to have 3 to 4 grams of carbohydrate per kilogram of body weight. If this recommendation feels like a lot of carbohydrate—or food in general—remember that you can always space it out a bit. For example, if you calculate your needs as approximately 250 grams of carbohydrate about four hours prior to activity, you could have closer to 175 grams in your pregame meal, then include another 75 grams slightly closer to competition.

Examples of Pregame Meals

- Omelet, toast, fruit, 2 slices turkey sausage, and orange juice
- Turkey and cheese sandwich, fruit, pretzels, and water
- Pasta with marinara sauce, chicken breast, broccoli, a breadstick, and water
- Sirloin steak, baked potato, roll, green beans, and water

As the training or competition gets closer, you move further down the funnel and room for flexibility with your nutrition choices narrows. The closer you get to competition, the leaner and more carbohydrate-rich your choices should be, and by the time you are an hour or less from the competition or training it is recommended to avoid protein and fat and choose primarily carbohydrates. This is not only because carbohydrates are your main energy source, but also because they are digested quickly and cause the least amount of GI distress. If you've ever experienced a practice or competition where you felt nauseous or like your pregame meal or snack wasn't sitting well, it's likely that you had too much fat or protein too close to activity and it wasn't digested completely.

As discussed in chapter 3, different types of carbohydrate can serve different purposes, depending on timing. Complex carbs have a higher fiber content, which makes them digest more slowly than simple carbohydrates. Although fiber is great to include in your diet, if you are an hour or less away from training or competition (at the bottom of the funnel), you should also try to limit high-fiber foods, which can cause gas, bloating, and GI discomfort. By this time, simple carbohydrates are recommended because they are quickly digested and can be an immediate energy source. You should aim for 1 to 2 grams of carbohydrate per kilogram of body weight if you are one to two hours out from activity. See table 3.1 in chapter 3 for examples of carb-rich foods, including simple carbohydrates.

In addition to carbohydrates, it is important to include fluids with your pregame meal and sip on hydrating fluids leading up to competition. This is especially important when consuming simple carbohydrates because without enough fluid, simple sugars can draw water into the stomach and cause fluid imbalances. Because the body can only process fluid so quickly, waiting until right before training or competition to drink a large volume of fluid will not adequately hydrate you. In addition, it will often cause GI distress—some athletes even feel a sloshing sensation when they drink too much fluid right before activity, which of course is uncomfortable and doesn't promote optimal performance. Hydrating fluids include water, flavored water, sports drinks, low-fat milk, tea, juice, protein shakes, and smoothies. The main fluids I would recommend you steer clear of in this time frame are soda and other carbonated drinks, energy drinks, and heavy coffee drinks (made with a lot of cream, for instance). More specific hydration recommendations are discussed in chapter 7.

Finally, it's common to have this pregame meal fall during breakfast, and many athletes struggle to eat much in the early morning. If that applies to you, I encourage you to prioritize carbohydrates and consider including carbohydrate-rich beverages like juice, milk, or smoothies, because it sometimes can be easier to drink something when you're not feeling especially hungry.

Intraworkout Nutrition

Perhaps not surprisingly, many of the same principles discussed in the immediate preworkout time frame apply once the workout or competition has started. During exercise your body reallocates blood flow to systems that need it most, namely skeletal muscles, and restricts blood flow to systems that are not vital to the process at hand, such as the GI tract. Because of this reduced blood flow, digestion is slowed significantly. It's for this reason that eating anything too heavy during a workout, especially protein, fat, or fiber, tends to cause GI distress like nausea and vomiting. During this time frame it's recommended to stick with simple

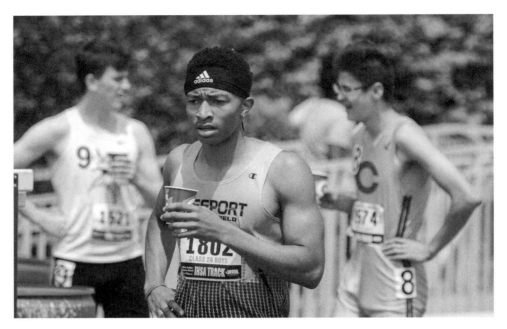

Carbohydrates are essential before, during, and after activity. Consuming them via sports drinks or other quick-digesting carbohydrates helps provide quick energy to boost performance.

carbohydrates, which are most easily digested and can be utilized as an immediate energy source.

How much carbohydrate you should aim to ingest during a workout depends on the type and length of activity. Refer back to the sidebar in chapter 3 for specific intraworkout carbohydrate recommendations.

Consider Logistics

Depending on the logistics of your sport, you may want to put in some thought into how you will consume food during the workout. Sports that have formal breaks like time-outs or halftime are fairly easy to navigate, and you can work snacks into these breaks. For sports that don't have realistic breaks worked into the existing rhythm—for example, endurance races—you may need to consider things that you can easily grab and consume on the go. Some good options could be carbohydrate gels or chews or packets of honey or applesauce. Sports drinks are also perfect for this scenario—they quickly and conveniently provide fluid, carbohydrates, and electrolytes. Other examples of logistical challenges include a sport like golf, where ideal options won't melt in the heat and can be consumed while walking the course, or cycling, where snacks need to be easily pulled out and consumed with one hand while not throwing off your balance or form.

Practice Beforehand

Whatever your situation, spend some time thinking about the unique challenges presented by your sport and environment and plan accordingly. Though it has been mentioned throughout this book, I can't stress enough how impactful it can be to practice your fueling strategy leading up to competition. Not only does practicing allow you to tweak your timing for fueling and hydration based on what you find improves performance the most, but it also allows you to experiment with different products, amounts, and even delivery methods. You might discover that using a gel instead of chews saves you some time and that you feel more energized or that certain products don't sit as well in your stomach. You can also work on training your body to handle larger amounts of fluid and carbohydrate if you are competing in endurance or ultraendurance sports and having a hard time meeting the recommended amounts. It can be effective to increase carbohydrate by 15 grams every couple of training sessions as you work up to the amounts that are recommended for your training.

Enlist Help

Depending on your resources and the level at which you're competing, you may also have a support team that helps track and deliver your fuel and hydration during competition. Although it may not be realistic to have your support team involved in all of your practice runs, you should involve them in the timing and fueling details that you have practiced leading up to the competition, if possible. They may be helpful in assisting in your fuel delivery plan in addition to tracking your intake amount and timing.

Considerations for Managing GI Discomfort

For some endurance sports, managing GI symptoms like nausea, bloating, or diarrhea is a crucial part of success. For sports that allow a more stationary position of the body during activity, like cycling and rowing, this tends to be less of a concern. Although adequate carbohydrate is still essential, athletes in these sports can afford the flexibility of a meal or snack closer to the workout as well as a little more fat at these times.

On the flip side, sports like running and swimming tend to cause jostling of the stomach (and its contents) and subsequently much more GI discomfort if fueling isn't carefully managed. Because of this risk, many athletes are fearful of eating in the time frame leading up to the workout or competition, which is detrimental to having enough carbohydrate on deck to fuel the workout itself, but also can make it challenging to get enough overall calories and carbohydrate if they avoid eating for long periods of time.

Causes of GI Discomfort

One of the most challenging aspects of managing GI discomfort is that there are a number of different causes, and they can be hard to pin down. There can be many unique responses to common causes of GI upset, and they tend to be inconsistent (something that upsets your stomach one day may not bother it the following week). Some common causes of GI symptoms include the following:

- *Diet.* Foods that are high in fat, fiber, or certain carbohydrates can trigger GI symptoms, and individuals can have negative responses to foods that they are sensitive to (e.g., lactose).
- *Dehydration.* Not getting enough fluid can lead to constipation or general digestive discomfort as a result of increased difficulty moving food through the GI system when there is not enough water in the gut.
- *Medications and supplements.* Some common medications like nonsteroidal anti-inflammatory drugs (NSAIDS) or antibiotics can irritate the GI tract and cause symptoms for some people. If you are using these medications habitually and you notice that you are frequently experiencing GI symptoms, you should discuss an alternative plan with your physician. Similarly, some supplement ingredients can cause GI symptoms, so if you have recently started taking a new supplement and start experiencing GI symptoms, discontinue the supplement and discuss with a physician or dietitian.
- *Stress and anxiety.* Mental health disturbances can often present themselves via GI symptoms in a number of different ways: Nausea, loss of appetite, diarrhea, and even constipation can all be a result of stress and anxiety, making this an important aspect of your health to manage.
- *Exercise.* Intense physical activity, especially for long amounts of time like endurance exercise requires, can divert blood flow away from the digestive system, causing symptoms like nausea, cramping, and diarrhea.
- *GI disorders.* Athletes are often victim to relatively common GI disorders such as gastroesophageal reflux disease (GERD), inflammatory bowel syndrome (IBS), ulcers, and more—which can cause both acute and chronic GI symptoms.

If you are experiencing abdominal pain or cramping, diarrhea, constipation, or bloating to the point of discomfort for more than a week at a time or many days of the week over a course of months, you should talk to a physician and a dietitian about what could be causing the symptoms. If you are experiencing any of these symptoms acutely, consider treating with over-the-counter medications and addressing any of the potential underlying causes mentioned previously, if possible.

Additionally, it's important that you do as much as you can to stay hydrated, especially if you are experiencing diarrhea or vomiting. Both of these symptoms cause increased water and electrolyte loss, so trying to replace as much of these lost fluids and nutrients as possible will be helpful in maintaining health and performance. In addition to just water you should consider including sports drinks with sodium, fruit, broth-based soups, and even popsicles or smoothies.

Proactive Strategies

Of course, some amount of GI discomfort here and there is normal and unavoidable—it's not uncommon for certain foods to cause a small amount of gas or bloating, and everyone will have the occasional misfortune of eating something that does not agree with their stomach. However, it is certainly in your best interest to do what you can to take a proactive approach to avoiding unwanted GI symptoms, especially leading up to and during activity.

Individualize Your Fueling

Remember the fueling strategies for the preworkout time frame discussed earlier in the chapter and the important role of carbohydrates, especially simple carbohydrates, at this time. Carbohydrates are digested more quickly, which reduces GI discomfort and allows the fuel source to be delivered more quickly to the muscles. Limit protein, fat, and fiber, which are digested more slowly and tend to cause GI symptoms. Also, be cognizant of foods that you know may cause you to experience any unpleasant symptoms. Although you shouldn't necessarily exclude a food because it bothered you one time, if you notice that a certain food or food group consistently bothers your stomach or causes any other symptoms, try to avoid these in your meals and snacks leading up to performance.

Control the Volume

The gut can be trained to tolerate higher volumes of liquids and even foods, though it takes time. If you struggle with GI symptoms during training, especially if it affects your ability take in enough calories or fluid, you should consider slowly working on increasing your tolerance to volume in your stomach. Start with a comfortable amount, and very slowly add just a little bit of volume at a time over your training days. Just as you would slowly work up your total mileage or training time, the same concept can apply here.

Stress and GI Symptoms

Stress and anxiety can be a common culprit of GI distress. It's not unusual for athletes to have some stress and anxiety, especially around competition, but anything you can do to manage stress could help manage those symptoms. Some athletes find they are successful in using breathing techniques, meditation, or simple yoga leading up to competition. Some physical therapists or coaches are trained specifically in breathing exercises and other techniques that could be helpful if you struggle with this aspect of your performance. Experiment with strategies that can help you relax and make those part of your routine—whether it's for training, competition, or both. If you find you cannot manage it on your own, consider working with a therapist or sport psychologist.

Postworkout Nutrition

As discussed briefly in the earlier chapters on carbohydrate and protein, athletes should never underestimate the importance of postworkout nutrition. Amidst busy schedules, the time frame after an athlete finishes a training session or competition can easily get consumed with other things, but research has solidly shown that proper nutrition in this time frame is important for many aspects of health and performance. It's not uncommon for athletes who are looking to get leaner to want to sacrifice the calories at this time, especially because they have often just finished burning a significant number of calories. However, this approach undermines an athlete's performance goals. On the contrary, athletes should prioritize this time and view it as an investment toward reaching their goals.

A postworkout meal or snack should include adequate calories and consist of both carbohydrate and protein, as well as fluid. I often refer to this approach as the *three Rs*: refuel, repair, and rehydrate.

Refuel

Include carbohydrate to replenish glycogen stores used during activity. It is recommended to consume 1 to 1.2 grams of carbohydrate per kilogram of body weight per hour for the first four hours following exercise.

Breaking this into small amounts of carbohydrate more frequently (every 15 to 30 minutes) may especially enhance this process, as can including high glycemic–index foods (mentioned in chapter 3). Although it may seem less practical, it may be worth the trouble for athletes participating in multiple training sessions per day or for dual-sport athletes who often have to quickly turn around and compete again.

Repair

Include protein to repair muscle proteins that were broken down during activity and promote MPS. As mentioned previously, there is some disparity in the research as to how much protein you need or how quickly you need it after a workout, but using the guidelines from chapter 4, you should take how much protein is recommended for your training and your body size and divide that across all your meals and snacks over the course of the day to determine how much protein to aim for in a postworkout snack. For most people that ends up being between 20 and 40 grams of protein. Similar to carbohydrate, it is advised to have another protein-rich meal or snack (20 to 40 grams) of protein an hour or two after that initial postworkout time frame. For most people this second dose correlates with having a meal. Ensuring this protein source is a complete protein, meaning it has all the essential amino acids, is best for stimulating MPS. Examples of these would include a protein shake or smoothie made with whey protein, meat, poultry, fish, eggs, Greek yogurt, milk, or soy milk. For more specifics on choosing a protein supplement, see chapter 8 on supplements.

Rehydrate

Include fluid to replace fluid lost during activity. It is recommended to consume 2 to 3 cups (16-24 fl oz) of fluid for every pound lost during exercise. As mentioned in chapter 7, it's not always realistic or necessary (or recommended) to weigh yourself for workouts, but if you have a hard time managing hydration you could consider taking pre- and post-workout weights to get an idea of your typical fluid loss and use that as a guide as you look to replace fluid. A more general recommendation is to drink to quench thirst after finishing activity, and then drink another 1 to 2 cups (8-16 fl oz).

There are plenty of great carbohydrate and protein combos for a postworkout meal listed in table 9.1. Some options naturally combine all of the three Rs by being a fluid as well as having protein and carbohydrate.

TABLE 9.1   Carb–Protein Combinations for Postworkout Fuel

Carbohydrate	Protein
Cereal	Milk
Bread	Lunch meat
Fruit	Jerky
Granola	Yogurt
Bagel	Peanut butter,
Crackers	Cheese
Toast	Hard boiled eggs
English muffin	Tuna
Bagel	Cottage cheese
Dried fruit	Nuts and seeds
ALL-IN-ONE FOODS	
Protein shakes with at least a 2-to-1 carb-to-protein ratio	Smoothies with protein powder, milk, or yogurt
Chocolate or strawberry milk	Protein bars

Making the Most of the Postworkout Window

Recommendations are usually for athletes to consume postworkout nutrition within 30 to 45 minutes of finishing exercise. For athletes who have to turn around and complete another workout or competition within 12 to 24 hours, this time frame is especially crucial. Although the total amount of carbohydrate and protein is most important, it may be useful to space it out over three to four hours after finishing, because smaller, more frequent amounts can increase absorption and utilization of both carbohydrate and protein. For athletes who are training just once per day, a more realistic approach might be having a postworkout snack, then following that with a balanced meal one to two hours later.

Effective postworkout fueling may take some planning. One common misstep among athletes is choosing not to grab postworkout fuel under the assumption that "I'm going to go eat right after this." The problem with this approach is that the time that elapses between finishing your activity and actually sitting down to eat can add up quickly. When you finish practice or training you likely cool down, stretch, and perhaps chat a little with coaches or teammates, then you probably shower, change, walk to your car, and drive home. Then, depending on what you're having, you may still need to cook when you get home or place an order when you get to the restaurant or dining hall. Ultimately, all of

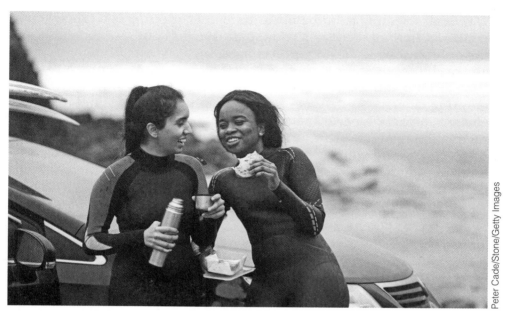

Peter Cade/Stone/Getty Images

Postworkout recovery should include both carbohydrate and protein but can come in many different forms, such as a premade beverage or snack bar, a freshly made smoothie, or even whole foods such as sandwiches.

these things can easily add up to over an hour or more—which means you've lost that window of efficient refueling. It's also not uncommon for athletes who don't plan ahead to get increasingly hungry following training, then end up settling for the quickest food they can get their hands on (like fast food), which often does not provide the most nutrient-dense option for recovery.

Evolving Fueling Needs

It's important to remember that although having a specific fueling plan is helpful to elicit a positive performance, it doesn't need to be set in stone. Fueling needs can ebb and flow based on a number of different factors. If you notice that you're training harder and feeling hungrier, it's totally reasonable to increase your fueling plan on those days. Similarly, the fueling needs of children and adolescents may vary a lot depending on whether they're currently going through a growth spurt—make sure to listen to hunger cues and respect that needs may be higher than estimated. Ultimately, your body is one of the best gauges of what it needs.

Overall, creating good habits around your training is a crucial component of finding success in your sport. Having solid fueling habits will not only pay dividends for performance, but also help promote recovery and overall health over time. Consider which aspects of pre-, intra-, and postworkout training you could improve, then work on slowly incorporating changes so that you can evaluate how you feel and take note of their impact on performance. Like so many aspects of performance fueling, be ready to pivot as your demands change and look for ways that you can individualize based on your preferences and needs. The following chapters will discuss different needs based on different kinds of training.

CHAPTER 10
Endurance Training and Competition

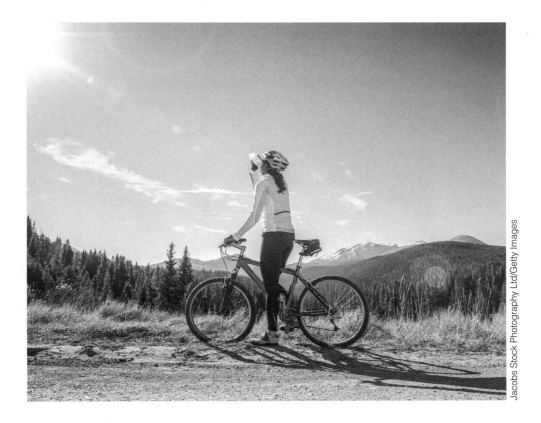

Jacobs Stock Photography Ltd/Getty Images

Endurance sports like long-distance running, swimming, cycling, and rowing have unique demands because their training requires not only a substantial amount of time, but also a very high energy expenditure. Unlike many skill-based sports, there tends to be less technical development and more of a focus on total volume of training. It is also common to train nearly year-round, so it is imperative to have good nutrition habits to support this consistently high energy expenditure. Although many other sports have an endurance component, this chapter will focus more specifically on activities lasting for two or more hours per day, such as running, swimming, cycling, and rowing.

Carbohydrate Needs

Foundational principles of fueling apply across the board to all sports; however, the high expenditure required for endurance sports makes adequate fueling vital—especially carbohydrate. If you think back to chapter 2, endurance training and competition are great examples of situations that would benefit from the plate in figure 2.3 showing half the plate dedicated to carbohydrates. This will help you keep up with the vast amount of carbohydrate that is required to fuel multiple hours of aerobic activity per day.

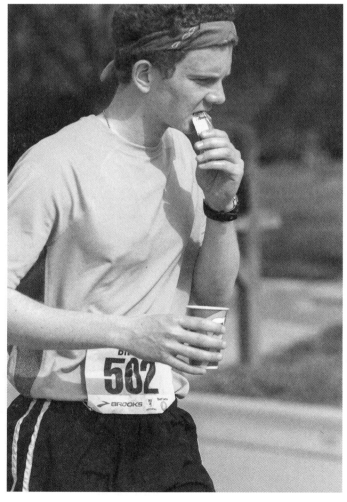

Quick-digesting carbohydrate sources like gels, chews, and sports drinks can help meet the high carbohydrate demands of endurance athletes.

TABLE 10.1   **Carbohydrate Recommendations for Endurance Training**

Type of activity	Recommended carbohydrate intake (g/kg)
Very light training (low-intensity or skill-based exercise)	3-5
Moderate-intensity training, 60 min/day	5-7
Moderate- to high-intensity endurance training, 1-3 hr/day	6-10
Moderate- to high-intensity endurance training, 4-5 hr/day	8-12

Chapter 3 discussed the different amount of carbohydrate needed based on volume of training. Table 10.1 shows these recommendations for endurance training. This refers to fairly intense training lasting an hour or more and may include sports that have an endurance component, like soccer, lacrosse, volleyball, basketball, and field hockey, as well as any classic endurance sport like running, swimming, cycling, or rowing—or, of course, any event that combines these activities, like triathlon.

Aiming to meet these higher carbohydrate recommendations tends to require very purposeful fueling that ensures each meal and snack contains adequate carbohydrate. Consult chapter 3 for a reminder of good sources of carbohydrate.

Protein Needs

Although carbohydrate is vital for an endurance athlete's success, it's important not to underestimate the role of protein. The importance of protein for endurance athletes has historically been downplayed, but more recent research has suggested that protein needs for endurance athletes may be higher than originally thought and might even be similar to those of strength and power athletes. Although the formal protein recommendation for endurance activity still tends to be 1.2 to 1.4 grams per kilogram per day, research has begun to show benefits for higher amounts in endurance athletes. Research by Kato and colleagues (2016) references the need for higher protein than is currently recommended, especially on training days. They recommended closer to 1.8 grams per kilogram on training days, with some research citing amounts as high as 2 grams per kilogram on training or competition days for ultraendurance athletes. Protein-rich foods are often a source of iron, a nutrient for which endurance athletes are more at risk of deficiency. Iron needs are discussed more in chapter 6.

Fat Needs

Although it doesn't garner as much attention, fat can be helpful for meeting the high energy expenditure associated with endurance training. In fact, consuming a diet that is too low in fat can make it incredibly hard to keep up with total energy needs. Trying to get adequate calories just from fruit, vegetables, protein, and whole grains can also lead to GI discomfort as a result of sheer volume, as well as the natural high fiber content of those foods. By including adequate fat in the diet, especially from foods high in healthy fats, it can help provide enough calories while controlling the total volume of food. Recommendations tend to be between 0.8 and 2 grams of fat per kilogram of body weight, depending on individual needs. Remember, however, that it is wise to limit fat leading up to training because of the increased likelihood of GI discomfort.

Medium-Chain Triglycerides (MCTs)

One kind of fat that is popular in endurance training specifically is medium-chain triglycerides (MCTs), a saturated fatty acid that has a shorter chemical structure than most other fats. MCTs are found in a variety of foods, though coconut and palm oil are the most well known. Although saturated fats are not usually recommended in general, MCTs have a few unique qualities that may make them appealing for endurance athletes. Their shorter chemical structure means they can be absorbed rapidly and converted into energy, making them a readily available fuel source, especially when glycogen is depleted toward the end of long-duration events. Their easy absorption also tends to make them well tolerated by the GI system, which is not the case for most fats. Although some endurance athletes may find these qualities to be helpful, a systemic review by Chapman-Lopez and Koh (2022) found that MCT oil showed very little to no ergogenic effect on exercise performance and macronutrient metabolism.

Low-Carbohydrate, High-Fat Diets

Although the ketogenic diet and its limitations have been discussed in previous chapters, it is a popular approach for endurance and ultraendurance athletes and should be addressed here. Research shows that adapting to a low-carbohydrate, high-fat (LCHF), or ketogenic, diet can lead to significant positive changes in how the body uses fat for energy during exercise, even in elite athletes who specifically train to optimize fat metabolism (Burke 2021). These changes typically occur within three to four weeks of following the diet, though Burke and colleagues (2021) found that in highly trained endurance athletes this can happen even more rapidly—as little as five to six days.

However, the effects of ketone use in muscles are still not fully understood, and there are unresolved questions about the ability to restore muscle glycogen levels. Keto-adaptation reduces the use of carbohydrates as fuel, and because the ability to utilize glycogen becomes important when oxygen supply is limited, this may have an impact on high-intensity exercise. The response to the LCHF diet can vary, with some athletes experiencing impaired performance and others benefiting from increased reliance on fat for energy. Athletes considering the ketogenic diet should weigh the potential benefits of fat utilization against the risk of impaired performance during high-intensity exercise due to limited carbohydrate availability. This is yet another example of the importance of trialing a fueling plan leading up to competition.

Hydration Needs

In addition to adequate macronutrients and overall calories, endurance athletes should also ensure adequate hydration and sodium replacement. Endurance athletes should be sure their hydration plan accounts for their individual sweat rate and includes sodium-rich beverages. See chapter 7 for more information on how to individualize your hydration plan.

Managing Weight

For better or worse, a common consideration for endurance athletes is managing weight. Although many athletes become very focused on weight, it's important to remember that there is no perfect body composition or weight for any athlete and that many things contribute far more to performance—including adequate sleep and nutrition, strength and conditioning, hydration, managing stress and anxiety, studying film, and skill development. With that said, when it comes to endurance sports like running, swimming, and cycling, it's reasonable to acknowledge that being lighter and having less mass to move across long distances can be beneficial.

It is important to understand that the relationship between weight and performance is not linear, but rather a bell-shaped curve. It is all too common for endurance athletes to lose a little bit of weight and notice that they cut a little bit of time off . . . so they strive to lose a little bit more. However, there is a point at which the weight loss is no longer beneficial: Being too lean can actually lead to decreased performance, GI problems, decreased bone health, stress fractures, and hormonal imbalances. Endurance athletes who are striving to decrease their weight should approach it slowly, during the off-season, while ensuring that they are fueling adequately and not affecting energy levels—females who notice menstrual cycle changes (they become lighter, irregular, or go away completely) are likely not fueling enough. You are encouraged to work with a registered dietitian if you are trying to manage weight goals and heavy training loads. See chapter 12 for more general tips on weight loss.

Fine-Tuning Your Fueling Routine

Although it is most important to establish solid foundational nutrition strategies, there are some more detail-oriented nutrition strategies that could further help you as an endurance athlete. For example, nitrates (discussed in chapter 8) can help increase blood flow to muscles and promote more efficient use of oxygen, which could give you that little bit of push down the stretch; many endurance athletes use beet juice for its high nitrate content.

Fighting Inflammation

Another strategy that you could consider is foods that have anti-inflammatory properties. Although most fruits, vegetables, and healthy fats have some anti-inflammatory effects, some in particular are especially popular among athletes, such as tart cherry juice. Although they can be helpful for any athlete, endurance athletes who do an immense amount of mileage—and therefore put an immense load on their joints—benefit from using tart cherry juices or concentrates with high antioxidant content to help fight inflammation during high workload time frames.

For similar reasons, omega-3 fatty acid supplementation can be advantageous to fight inflammation. The most common omega-3 fatty acid supplement is fish oil. In addition to the normal supplement considerations discussed in chapter 8, you should look for one that has about a 2-to-1 EPA to DHA ratio.

Carbohydrate Loading

As mentioned in chapter 3, carbohydrate loading can be an effective strategy for endurance athletes, but it should be approached strategically. A common misconception about carbohydrate loading is that it's as simple as eating a couple of platefuls of pasta the night before a big race. However, it is more involved than that and takes a thoughtful approach. The most recent recommendations outlined in table 10.2 suggest that athletes should rest for 36 to 48 hours and consume 10 to 12 grams of

TABLE 10.2   Carbohydrate Loading Recommendations

Day	Training	Carbohydrate
1	Rest	10-12 g/kg
2	Rest	10-12 g/kg
3	Competition	Follow carbohydrate guidelines for before, during, and after competition

carbohydrate per kilogram per day in the 24 to 48 hours leading up to competition day. Fairchild and colleagues (2002) specifically found that such protocols could result in a near doubling of muscle glycogen concentrations. One important consideration brought up by Wismann and Willoughby (2006) is the differences in carbohydrate loading for women as compared to men. Women were able to achieve the same results as men when taking in comparable amounts of carbohydrate relative to lean body mass; however, women may need to significantly increase their total caloric intake over the loading days to achieve these results.

Getting this high amount of carbohydrate will likely require eating frequently throughout the day. Athletes may find more success in choosing low-fiber foods like white pasta, white rice, bread, simple cereals, fruit, granola bars, lower-fat baked goods and desserts, yogurt, milk, and sports

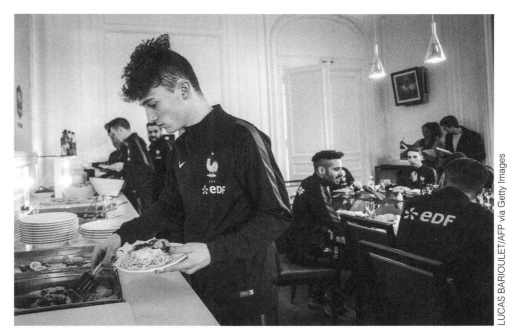

LUCAS BARIOULET/AFP via Getty Images

Carbohydrate loading is a popular approach for endurance athletes, but is often misunderstood. Carbohydrate loading involves eating extra carbohydrate for not just one day, but the three days leading up to competition.

drinks, gels, and chews. As for any competition day regimen, make sure you practice this fueling technique prior to competition and ensure that you have a plan in place that works for you and does not cause GI upset!

Competition

Many of the principles of fueling before, during, and after competition discussed in chapter 9 apply to endurance competitions as well. Revisit those suggestions when creating a nutrition plan to ensure adequate carbohydrate intake and avoid GI upset. Because endurance events, especially ones that take many hours to complete, tend to start in the morning, your competition day plan should start the day or two leading up to the event.

Two sample fueling plans for endurance athletes are shown next. The first plan (Athlete 1 Sample Fuel Plan) supports a 125-pound (56.8 kg) female athlete for a three-hour marathon starting at 8 a.m. and uses a recommendation of 8 grams per kilogram of carbohydrate, which is on the low end for endurance athletes at this intensity and duration. Remember that for endurance competitions lasting two to three hours, the goal is to have 60 grams of carbohydrate every hour to keep up with needs.

Athlete 1 Sample Fuel Plan

This fuel plan is based on 454 grams of carbohydrate per day (56.8 kg × 8 g/kg), which could be divided across three meals of approximately 120 grams each and two snacks of approximately 55 grams each. It is not an exact science, though, and can be divided up however it makes sense for your schedule, as long as you are aiming to get the total number. It's important to note that carbohydrate recommendations like the one above (8g/kg/d) are designed to support your everyday training and energy needs. Competition days, especially for endurance sports where you cover significantly more mileage than in training days, will inherently require more carbohydrate. While meals and snacks should look generally similar, intracompetition fueling will put your carbohydrate total for the day significantly higher.

NIGHT BEFORE COMPETITION

Dinner (6 p.m.)

2 cups pasta, 1 cup marinara sauce, 1 oz mozzarella cheese, 4 oz grilled chicken breast (with salt and pepper), 1 cup green beans (120 g CHO, 40 g PRO, 20 g FAT)

Late night snack (9 p.m.)

5 oz Greek yogurt, 1/2 cup berries, 1/2 cup granola (55 g CHO, 15 g PRO, 15 g FAT)

DAY OF COMPETITION

Breakfast (5 a.m.)

2 scrambled eggs (with salt), 3 pancakes (6 in. diameter), 4 tbsp maple syrup, 8 fl oz orange juice, 16 fl oz water (150 g CHO, 30 g PRO, 35 g FAT)

Precompetition snack (7:30 a.m.)

1 oz pretzels, 8 fl oz sports drink, 8 fl oz water (30 g CHO, 2 g PRO, 1 g FAT)

170 grams of carbohydrate are needed three hours out from competition (56.8 kg × 3 g/kg). 150 grams were allotted at the prerace meal, and the rest was included in a precompetition snack to help space it out.

Race begins (8 a.m.)

Aim for ~60 g/hr CHO during race

Hydration stop (8:30 a.m.)

8 fl oz water

Snack 1 (9 a.m.)

1 sports gel, 12 fl oz sports drink (50 g CHO)

Hydration stop (9:30 a.m.)

8 fl oz sports drink (15 g CHO)

Snack 2 (10 a.m.)

12 fl oz sports drink, 6 sports chews (45 g CHO)

Hydration stop (10:30 a.m.)

8 fl oz sports drink (15 g CHO)

Race ends (11 a.m.)

16-24 fl oz water (or more if you are a heavy sweater)

Postworkout snack

Ready-to-drink protein shake (40 g CHO, 20 g PRO, 1 g FAT)

Lunch (2 p.m.)

Grilled chicken wrap with cheese, veggies, and mayo (35 g CHO, 40 g PRO, 20 g FAT)

Dinner (6 p.m.)

2 cups orzo, 4 oz salmon, 1 cup broccoli, 1 cup watermelon, 1 dinner roll, 1 Tbsp butter (115 g CHO, 43 g PRO, 25 g FAT)

Late night snack (9 p.m.)

1 cup Greek yogurt, ¼ cup granola, ½ cup berries (45 g CHO, 12 g PRO, 8 g FAT)

56.8 grams of postworkout carbohydrate are needed (56.8 kg × 1 g/kg). Aim to include most of this in postworkout snack and the remaining amount in lunch a couple of hours later.

The second sample fueling plan is designed to support a 165-pound (75 kg) male athlete for a three-hour triathlon starting at 12 p.m. This example uses a recommendation of 10 grams per kilogram of carbohydrate per day.

Athlete 2 Sample Fuel Plan

This fuel plan is based on 750 grams of carbohydrate per day (75 kg × 10 g/kg). This could be divided across three meals of approximately 150 grams each and four snacks of approximately 75 grams each. This does not need to be exact and can be divided up however it makes sense for your schedule, as long as you are aiming to get the total number. Remember too that on a competition day, the total carbohydrate will be higher than the recommendation above. That recommendation is designed to support your normal training and everyday needs.

NIGHT BEFORE COMPETITION

Dinner (6 p.m.)

3 cups pasta, 1 cup marinara sauce, 1 oz mozzarella cheese, 6 oz grilled chicken breast (with salt and pepper), 1 cup green beans, 1 breadstick (150 g CHO, 80 g PRO, 20 g FAT)

Late night snack (9 p.m.)

2 cups Honey Nut Cheerios, 12 fl oz milk (75 g CHO, 20 g PRO, 8 g FAT)

DAY OF COMPETITION

Breakfast (8 a.m.)

3 scrambled eggs (with salt), 3 slices white toast, 4 tbsp jam, 2 cups oatmeal, 2 tbsp honey, 1 cup fresh berries (225 g CHO, 35 g PRO, 20 g FAT)

Precompetition snack (11 a.m.)

1 banana, 1/2 bagel, 1 tbsp jam, 12-16 fl oz water (70 g CHO, 8 g PRO, 1 g FAT)

300 grams of carbohydrate are needed four hours out from competition (75 kg × 4 g/kg). 225 grams were allotted at the prerace meal, and the other 70 were included in a precompetition snack to help space it out.

Race begins (12 p.m.)

Aim for ~60 g/hr CHO during the race

Hydration and transition (12:30 p.m.)

8 fl oz sports drink (15 g CHO)

Snack 1 (on bike) (1 p.m.)

1 applesauce pouch, 12 fl oz sports drink (40 g CHO)

Snack 2 and transition (1:45 p.m.)

2 fl oz sports drink, 6 sports chews (45 g CHO)

Hydration (2:15 p.m.)

12 fl oz sports drink (22 g CHO)

Hydration (2:30 p.m.)

8 fl oz sports drink (15 g CHO)

Race ends (3 p.m.)

16-24 fl oz water (or more depending on sweat rate)

Postworkout snack (3:30 p.m.)

Ready-to-drink protein shake (40 g CHO, 20 g PRO, 1 g FAT)

Dinner (5:30 p.m.)

2 cups rice, 6 oz chicken, 1 cup mixed vegetables, 1/2 cup teriyaki sauce (115 g CHO, 50 g PRO, 5 g FAT)

Late night snack (9:30 p.m.)

1.5 cups Cheerios, 1 cup 2% milk (46 g CHO, 18 g PRO, 8 g FAT)

75 grams of postworkout carbohydrate are needed (75 kg × 1 g/kg). Aim to include most of this in a postworkout snack and hit the remaining amount during dinner a couple of hours later.

Bringing It All Together

These are just examples of meal plans that can support the high needs of an endurance athlete on competition day. Your fueling plan should account for your body size, needs, preferences, and what you've found to work for you during training. I would also encourage you to think about any logistical challenges that might come up. If you're competing in an unfamiliar town, do your research and find what food options are available nearby. There are often plenty of good options that can be found at restaurants (pasta, sandwiches, stir fry, etc.), but remember that you should stick to things you know don't upset your stomach and be very sure that the food is prepared in a safe manner. If you are concerned about this, you might be better off going to a grocery store or packing foods that you can prepare in a hotel room that will still meet your needs. If you choose to go this route, call ahead to see what is available at the hotel in terms of access to a fridge or microwave—this could dictate your plan.

Finally, do what you can to not stress. Although it's often hard to avoid completely when the big competition comes around, stress and anxiety can cause a whole host of side effects that can be detrimental to performance, including increased heart rate and respiration, GI distress, and increased perceived exertion. Having practiced your fueling plan and feeling confident in that aspect of your routine can help relieve some of that stress and anxiety. In addition, you can practice other methods of relaxation like yoga, meditation, listening to music, and breathing exercises—there are a number of apps available that can help with stress management. Ultimately, the more you can try to control the things you can control and let go of the rest, the more likely you will be to capitalize on the training you've put in and have a good race.

Fueling endurance activity requires an immense amount of calories and a purposeful approach to where those calories come from. Ensuring that you are eating enough carbohydrate and timing the intake appropriately before and during training and competition can make a significant difference in performance. Especially given how much time is often spent training for these endurance events, it makes sense to want to maximize your efforts and ensure that your hard work and commitment pays off!

CHAPTER 11

Strength, Power, and Team Sport Training and Competition

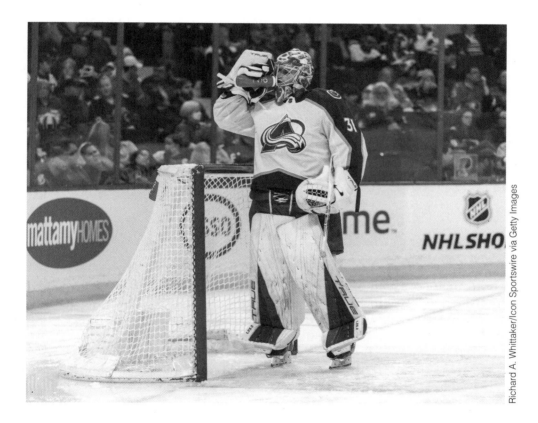

Richard A. Whittaker/Icon Sportswire via Getty Images

Although many aspects of training and competition for strength and power sports are similar to other sports, there are also many key differences. Though of course the exact extent to which athletes use the different energy systems varies widely based on sport (and in some cases by individual athlete and position), strength and power athletes rely heavily on the anaerobic systems (immediately available energy, does not utilize oxygen), whereas endurance athletes rely mostly on the aerobic system (more slowly utilized and therefore able to use oxygen). This chapter will discuss training and competition considerations for strength, power, and team sports. Each sport in this category involves a combination of strength, speed, explosiveness, and endurance, and most involve at least some degree of technical skill. Although leanness could be beneficial for some aspects of performance in these sports, more often an emphasis is put on building muscle and subsequently strength and power.

Although endurance sports rely heavily on adequate carbohydrate, it's important to remember that quick, explosive movements are also fueled primarily by carbohydrate, so adequate fueling before training and competition is still essential for power and strength athletes. Generally speaking, the amount of total carbohydrate needed over the course of a day tends to be lower than that needed by endurance and ultraendurance athletes, but strength and power athletes should still aim to consistently include carbohydrate throughout the day to ensure that they have adequate fuel available to support training needs. Many athletes training for strength, power, and team sports may have needs that are represented by the baseline plate in figure 2.2 (equal thirds of carbohydrate, protein, and fruit and vegetables). However, this category represents a wide variety of sports and situations, so it's important to think about your training when determining what might be best for you. Carbohydrate needs for light- to moderate-intensity sports are shown in table 11.1.

Carbohydrate Needs

Some team sports, such as soccer and lacrosse, do have a significant endurance component. If you train in one of these sports, your carbohydrate needs are likely closer to 6 to 10 grams per kilogram per day, or half your plate from carbohydrate—especially if training loads are high, you are playing a lot of minutes, or you compete in tournaments with quick turnaround of games.

Many team sports have an endurance component but are predominantly characterized by power, speed, and explosiveness. Examples of these would be football, basketball, volleyball, gymnastics, wrestling, tennis, and track (middle distance). Although endurance is not always highlighted, many of these sports can situationally become very endurance-heavy—for example, volleyball going five sets or a basketball game going into overtime. In these situations, athletes must be able to continue to produce fast, explosive movements again and again despite being fatigued. The recommended carbohydrate intake for athletes in these sports would likely fall anywhere between 5 and 10 grams per kilogram per day depending on the training and the season.

There are also many sports that rely primarily on technical skill and very short bouts of strength and explosiveness—for example, baseball,

TABLE 11.1 Carbohydrate Recommendations for Strength, Power, and Team Sport Training

Type of activity	Recommended carbohydrate intake (g/kg)	Portion sizes
Very light (low-intensity or skill-based) training	3–5	
Moderate-intensity training, 60 min/day	5–7	
Moderate- to high-intensity endurance exercise, 1–3 hr/day	6–10	
Moderate- to high-intensity exercise, 4–5 hr/day	8–12	

Reprinted by permission from L. Link, *The Healthy Former Athlete* (New York: Skyhorse Publishing, 2018).

softball, track (sprints, jumps, throws), diving, and golf. Consequently, these sports are relatively low in terms of the carbohydrate needed to fuel them. These athletes still need carbohydrate, but less than the examples that have been covered up to this point. Although there may be exceptions during very high training periods, generally carbohydrate needs are between 3 and 5 grams per kilogram per day, or about one-fourth of a plate comprising carbohydrate.

Another important thing to note about sports with lower overall carbohydrate requirements is that these sports rarely need the significant amounts of carbohydrate that are usually recommended leading up to activity (the 4, 3, 2, 1 rule discussed in chapter 3). Although these athletes still need carbohydrate in their pregame meal, they can approach it just like they would any other meal and aim to spread their daily carbohydrate needs spread over their meals and snacks for the day.

Protein Needs

Protein is important for any athlete, but for athletes trying to build lean muscle mass and improve strength, power, and explosiveness, it is vital. The recommendation for athletes partaking in anaerobic training is between 1.4 and 2 grams per kilogram of protein per day. This should be spread out over the entire day. It's a common misconception that more protein automatically equals more muscle and especially common for athletes in strength and power sports to eat one or two meals that are practically all protein. As discussed in chapter 4, total protein intake is important, but the most important factor in protein consumption is regular and consistent protein intake—periods of elevated MPS should occur multiple times, and this consistent intake provides a regular stimulus for MPS.

Fat Needs

There are no specific recommendations in regards to fat for team, power, and strength sports. Athletes competing in these sports should aim to follow the general recommendations of getting 20 to 35 percent of total calories from fat. For athletes competing in these sports who have a very high expenditure or are trying to gain or maintain weight, aiming for the high end of this range may be beneficial in trying to keep caloric intake high without feeling overly full.

Hydration Needs

In addition to adequate macronutrients and overall calories, athletes in power, strength, and team sports should also ensure adequate hydration. Athletes should have a hydration plan that accounts for their individual sweat rate and include sodium-rich beverages if needed. For a sport like football, for instance, the pads and helmet tend to contribute to a higher-than-average sweat rate. On the other hand, sports that are mostly skill based may lend themselves to a very low sweat rate, in which case sodium-rich beverages are likely not needed. See chapter 7 for more information on how to individualize your hydration plan.

No One Size Fits All

One of the trickier parts of being a team sport athlete is that there are often many different positions, each with different roles that can lend themselves to different body types and call for different skill sets. Football is perhaps one of the most dramatic examples of this (though far from

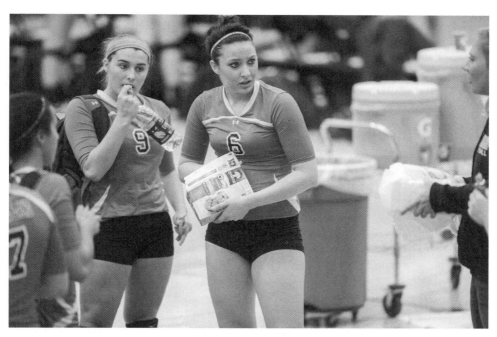

It can sometimes be hard to meet individual nutritional needs on a team with many athletes. Plan ahead to ensure that you can structure your fueling program around training and competition.

the only one). Lineman need to be strong and explosive as well as carry a lot of mass. Wide receivers need to be lean and fast. Running backs need to be strong, fast, and agile. It would be ridiculous to assume that all of these different players should be eating and fueling the exact same way with their different requirements and body types—yet it can be easy to look around and compare yourself to teammates or find yourself feeling like you should be eating the same way they do. Don't get caught in this trap! Your fueling needs are unique to you and your body, your sport, your position, and your goals.

Fine-Tuning Your Fueling Routine

As mentioned at the beginning of this chapter, leanness can be beneficial for some strength and power athletes, but these athletes are often more focused on gaining lean mass and promoting overall strength. For some sports like football, this goal may be very weight oriented. It's important to approach any weight or body composition goal safely and evaluate yourself and your performance as you go. As I often remind athletes I work with, if you feel terrible and play terrible, it doesn't matter what your weight is. Focus first on performance, and then on weight if necessary. Basic guidelines for safe weight gain and loss are discussed in chapter 12, but if you are trying to change weight drastically or if you participate in a weight-class sport like wrestling, boxing, rowing, or any of the martial arts, I would strongly encourage you to work with a registered dietitian who could help you approach your goal safely and with your health and performance in mind.

Fighting Inflammation

Although focusing on foundational nutrition strategies first is crucial, there are more specific nutrition strategies that can further benefit you as a strength, power, or team sport athlete, such as foods with anti-inflammatory properties. Tart cherry juice is one such popular option because it contains high levels of antioxidants and has anti-inflammatory effects. Although they can be beneficial for any athlete, those who put significant stress on their joints, particularly involving repetitive motions (e.g., baseball pitchers, offensive linemen, throwers, and jumpers), can benefit from incorporating tart cherry juices or concentrates into their routine during intense training periods. The timing of consuming tart cherry juice isn't as important as using it consistently during high workload periods.

For similar reasons, omega-3 fatty acid supplementation can be advantageous to fight inflammation. Fish oil is the most common form of omega-3 fatty acid supplement. Consider the information discussed in chapter 8 about choosing supplements, and look for one with an EPA-to-DHA ratio of approximately 2-to-1. There is no specific time of day that is perfect for taking omega-3s; as with tart cherry juice, the key is to take it regularly.

Creatine

Creatine is also popular among strength and power athletes, and it's easy to understand why: Supplemental creatine has been shown to increase strength and power and improve overall maximal effort. It can also be helpful when trying to increase mass and gain weight. There are a number of forms of creatine available on the market; however, 100 percent creatine monohydrate is the most widely used and studied form of creatine in supplements and the one I would recommend. More information on creatine and dosing can be found in chapter 8.

Competition

Many of the principles around pre-, inter-, and postcompetition nutrition discussed in chapter 9 apply to power, strength, and team sport competitions as well. Consider these recommendations when formulating

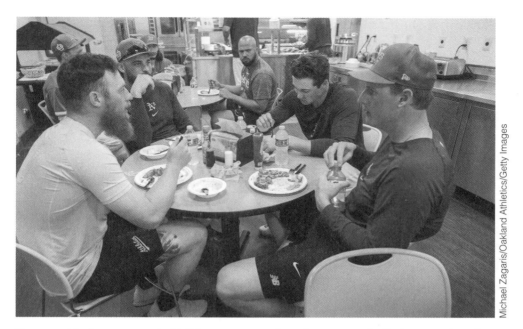

Use provided resources to build pregame and postgame meals that support performance and your unique needs.

your competition plan, and strive for a well-rounded, moderately low-fat pregame meal. It's crucial to select foods that you are familiar with and that do not cause stomach discomfort. For sports that do not involve a lot of jostling of the stomach or require prolonged endurance, you might be able to have a slightly more substantial meal. However, regardless of your sport, it is essential to test your competition day fueling plan before the actual event.

The following are some examples of competition fueling plans for strength, power, or team sport athletes. Although many different examples of fueling plans could be used, these will provide a framework of what such a plan might look like. The first sample plan is for a male diver who weighs 150 pounds (68.18 kg), using a carbohydrate recommendation of 4 grams per kilogram per day. The diving competition begins at 11 a.m.

Athlete 1 Sample Fuel Plan

As mentioned earlier in the chapter, there is no need to follow the 4, 3, 2, 1 recommendation for technical or skill-based sports with low overall carbohydrate requirements. Instead, focus on including carbohydrate in your meals like you typically would—by spreading your daily carbohydrate recommendation over your meals and snacks for the day. In this case, 273 grams of carbohydrate (68.18 kg × 4 g/kg) could be spread over three meals of 68 grams each and two snacks of 34 grams each.

(continued)

Athlete 1 Sample Fuel Plan *(continued)*

BEFORE THE COMPETITION

Breakfast (8 a.m.)

2 scrambled eggs, 1.5 cups oatmeal, 1/2 cup blueberries, 1 tbsp peanut butter, 16 fl oz water (57 g CHO, 26 g PRO, 22 g FAT)

Preworkout snack (10:30 a.m.)

1 banana, 12 fl oz water (28 g CHO, 1 g PRO)

DURING THE COMPETITION

Competition begins (11 a.m.)

Aim for ~15 g/hr CHO during competition

Snack 1 (1:30 p.m.)

8 fl oz water, 8 fl oz Gatorade (15 g CHO)

Snack 2 (2:30 p.m.)

1 oz pretzels, 8 fl oz water (23 g CHO, 3 g PRO, 1 g FAT)

AFTER THE COMPETITION

Postworkout snack (2:30 p.m.)

Ready-to-drink protein shake (20 g CHO, 20 g PRO, 1 g FAT)

Lunch (3:30 p.m.)

Grilled chicken wrap with cheese, veggies, and mayo (35 g CHO, 40 g PRO, 20 g FAT)

Dinner (7 p.m.)

6 oz salmon, 1 cup wild rice, 1 cup asparagus (55 g CHO, 45 g PRO, 22 g FAT)

Late night snack (9 p.m.)

1 Greek yogurt (5.3 oz cup), 1/2 cup strawberries, 2 cups popcorn (35 g CHO, 15 g PRO, 1 g FAT)

Approximately 68 grams of postworkout carbohydrate are needed (68.18 kg × 1 g/kg). For athletes in lower-expenditure sports that use less glycogen, this can be spread between the postworkout snack and the following meal.

The next fueling plan is for a 180-pound (81.8 kg) female volleyball player whose match begins at 8 p.m. This example uses a recommendation of 7 grams per kilogram of carbohydrate per day. Keep in mind that for sports that have an endurance component, competition days might require higher carbohydrate than training days to reflect the higher energy needs on a game day—especially if the competition runs long for any reason.

Athlete 2 Sample Fuel Plan

This fuel plan is based on 573 grams of carbohydrate a day (81.8 kg × 7 g/kg). This could be divided across four meals of approximately 100 grams each and three snacks of approximately 55 grams each. This does not need to be exact and can be divided up however it makes sense for your schedule, as long as you are aiming to get the total number.

BEFORE THE MATCH

Breakfast (9 a.m.)

3 scrambled eggs (with salt), 2 turkey sausage links, 2 slices French toast, 4 tbsp maple syrup, 1 cup mixed berries (100 g CHO, 35 PRO, 30 g FAT)

Lunch (12:30 p.m.)

8-in. sub sandwich with turkey, cheese, veggies, and mayo, 1 oz baked chips, 1 large dill pickle, 1 banana (105 g CHO, 30 g PRO, 25 g FAT)

Pregame meal (4 p.m.)

3 cups pasta, 1 cup marinara, 4 oz chicken breast, 2 cups spinach salad, 2 tbsp Italian dressing, 12 fl oz sports drink (170 g CHO, 55 g PRO, 13 g FAT)

Pregame snack (7:30 p.m.)

1 Chewy granola bar, 12 fl oz sports drink (42 g CHO, 1 g PRO, 3 g FAT)

246 grams of carbohydrate are needed three hours out from competition (81.8 kg × 3 g/kg). Approximately 170 grams were allotted at the pregame meal, and another 40 grams were included in a pregame snack to help space it out.

DURING THE MATCH

Match starts (8 p.m.)

Aim for ~30 g/hr CHO during the match

Hydration (after set 1)

16-24 fl oz water (or more depending on sweat rate)

Snack (after set 2)

12 fl oz sports drink, 6 sports chews (45 g CHO)

Hydration (after set 3)

16-24 fl oz water (or more depending on sweat rate)

Snack (after set 4 if needed)

12 oz sports drink (22 g CHO)

(continued)

Athlete 2 Sample Fuel Plan   *(continued)*

AFTER THE MATCH

Postworkout snack (10:30 p.m.)

Ready-to-drink protein shake (40 g CHO, 20 g PRO, 1 g FAT)

Dinner (11:00 p.m.)

1.5 cups rice, 6 oz chicken, 1 cup mixed vegetables, 3 tbsp teriyaki sauce (90 g CHO, 75 g PRO, 20 g FAT)

Approximately 81 grams of postworkout carbohydrate are needed (81.2 kg × 1 g/kg). Aim to include some of this in a postworkout snack and any remaining amount in dinner afterward. It can be challenging to meet postworkout nutrition needs before going to bed after late night competitions, but it is essential. If a meal doesn't seem realistic, consider having a couple of ready-to-drink shakes or a smoothie—it can sometimes be easier to drink something than to eat.

The next sample fuel plan is for a 285-pound (129.5 kg) male football player playing at 3:30 p.m. This example uses a recommendation of 6 grams per kilogram of carbohydrate per day. Keep in mind that a sport like football does have an endurance component due to the long game time (typically over four hours). As such, game days might require higher amounts of carbohydrate than practice days to reflect the higher energy needs on a game day.

Athlete 3 Sample Fuel Plan

This fuel plan is based on 777 grams of carbohydrate a day (129.5 kg × 6 g/kg). This could be divided across four meals of approximately 150 grams each and two snacks of approximately 75 grams each. This does not need to be exact and can be divided up however it makes sense for your schedule, as long as you are aiming to get the total number.

BEFORE THE GAME

Breakfast (9 a.m.)

3-egg omelet with veggies, 1 bagel, 2 tbsp cream cheese, 1 banana, 8 fl oz orange juice (110 g CHO, 40 g PRO, 25 g FAT)

Lunch (pregame meal) (12 p.m.)

4 cups pasta, 1.5 cups marinara, 5 oz chicken breast, 1/2 cup broccoli, 1 breadstick, 16 fl oz sweet tea (240 g CHO, 80 g PRO, 15 g FAT)

Pregame snack (3 p.m.)

1 Chewy granola bar, 1/2 cup dried fruit, 20 fl oz sports drink (80 g CHO, 2 g PRO, 3 g FAT)

Approximately 388 grams of carbohydrate are needed three hours out from competition (129.5 kg × 3 g/kg). 240 grams were allotted at the pregame meal (lunch), and the rest was included in a pregame snack to help space it out. Aim for 15-30 g/CHO/hr. Football is a very long duration sport with intermittent intensity, so this range proves to be sufficient for most players.

DURING THE GAME

Game starts (3:30 p.m.)

Aim for 15-30 g/hr CHO during the game (though football games are long in duration, the intensity is intermittent, so this range proves to be sufficient for most players)

Snack 1 (during first quarter)

16 fl oz water, 8 fl oz sports drink (15 g CHO)

Snack 2 (during second quarter)

8 fl oz sports drink (15 g CHO)

Snack 3 (halftime)

Peanut butter and jelly sandwich (60 g CHO, 15 g PRO, 20 g FAT)

Snack 4 (during third quarter)

16 fl oz water, 8 fl oz sports drink (15 g CHO)

Snack 5 (during fourth quarter)

6 sports chews (24 g CHO)

AFTER THE GAME

Postworkout snack (7 p.m.)

Ready-to-drink protein shake, 8 fl oz cherry juice (70 g CHO, 20 g PRO, 1 g FAT)

Dinner (8 p.m.)

Steak burrito (rice, beans, steak, cheese, veggies), guacamole, tortilla chips (150 g CHO, 45 g PRO, 35 g FAT)

Late night snack (10 p.m.)

2 cups Honey Bunches of Oats cereal, 2 cups milk, 1 banana (130 g CHO, 15 g PRO, 5 g FAT)

Approximately 130 grams of postworkout carbohydrate are needed (129.5 kg × 1 g/kg). Aim to include some of this in a postworkout snack and any remaining amount in dinner afterward.

The last fuel plan presented is for a 140-pound (63.50 kg) female soccer player participating in a 6:00 a.m. workout during off-season training. This example uses a recommendation of 7 grams per kilogram of carbohydrate per day.

Athlete 4 Sample Fuel Plan

This fuel plan is based on 445 grams of carbohydrate per day (63.6 kg × 7 g/kg). This could be divided across three meals of approximately 100 grams each and four snacks of approximately 35 grams each. This does not need to be exact and can be divided up however it makes sense for your schedule, as long as you are aiming to get the total number.

BEFORE TRAINING

Preworkout snack (5:30 a.m.)

1 applesauce pouch, 8 fl oz sports drink, 8 fl oz orange juice (35 g CHO, 1 g PRO)

Approximately 64 grams of carbohydrate are needed one hour or less from training (63.6 kg × 1 g/kg). The sample preworkout snack included closer to half of this amount—because many athletes don't want to wake up earlier than necessary for early morning workouts, this snack was eaten only 30 minutes out.

AFTER TRAINING

Postworkout snack (7:30 a.m.)

16 fl oz chocolate milk (38 g CHO, 16 g PRO, 5 g FAT)

Breakfast (8 a.m.)

2 slices wheat bread, 2 scrambled eggs, 1/2 sliced avocado, 2 tbsp jam (100 g CHO, 40 g PRO, 28 g FAT)

Lunch (12:30 p.m.)

5 oz chicken breast, 1.5 cups quinoa, 1 cup mixed veggies, 1 cup berries (90 g CHO, 60 g PRO, 11 g FAT)

Afternoon snack (7 p.m.)

1 banana, 1 tbsp peanut butter, 1 string cheese (40 g CHO, 12 g PRO, 14 g FAT)

Dinner (8 p.m.)

4 oz salmon, 1 large sweet potato, 1 tbsp butter, 2 tbsp brown sugar, 1 cup Brussels sprouts, 1 cup watermelon (90 g CHO, 35 g PRO, 15 g FAT)

Late night snack (10 p.m.)

6-8 crackers, 2 oz Colby jack cheese, 1 kiwi (37 g CHO, 18 g PRO, 10 g FAT)

Bringing It All Together

One challenge for team sport athletes specifically is that you may be at the mercy of what your team plans for pre- and postgame meals. You may not have complete control, but there are a couple of things you can try if you are unable to choose the menu or location. You might consider talking to the coach or staff member in charge of planning to explain the importance of making purposeful pre- and postgame nutrition choices. You might also request that certain foods that work well for you be made available, especially in the pregame time frame. Remember, though, that your coach is balancing the needs of the entire group, so be realistic about the logistics and budget. Ultimately, you should do whatever you can to get the needed amount of carbohydrate and protein, particularly carbohydrate. In the absence of a food allergy or intolerance, there is no good excuse to skip a pre- or postgame meal. You should view these meals as an important part of your performance—just like you wouldn't skip weights just because you didn't love the equipment in the weight room, you shouldn't skip a meal just because it's not your preferred food choice. At the end of the day, if the coach or staff are unable to accommodate you and you truly feel like there are not appropriate options for you, consider planning ahead and packing something for these meals.

Finally, make an effort to minimize stress as much as possible. Although it may be challenging to completely avoid stress during competitions, it's important to recognize that stress and anxiety can have negative effects on performance, including elevated heart rate and respiration, GI discomfort, and heightened perception of exertion. For some individuals, feeling confident in their practiced fueling plan can help alleviate some of this stress and anxiety. You can try sipping on ginger ale or taking over-the-counter stomach medication to help alleviate any GI discomfort. Additionally, incorporating relaxation techniques like yoga, meditation, listening to music, and breathing exercises can be beneficial—numerous apps are available that can help with stress management. You can also lean on teammates or trusted coaches and support staff if that helps to ease any stress or anxiety you might be feeling. The more you are able to do this, the greater your chances of capitalizing on your training and performing at your best.

Because strength, power, and team sports encompass a vast range of athletics—and often a vast number of positions and situations within each sport—it can be difficult to pin down recommendations that are specific to your needs. For this reason, it is incredibly helpful to be as tuned in as possible to how you are feeling and performing as you make changes to your nutrition plan. When evaluating your macronutrient needs, for instance, start in the middle and evaluate your energy levels, hunger cues, and whether you are progressing toward your goals (conditioning and strength, weight, etc.). If you feel like you energy levels are low, you're hungry all the time, your performance is suffering, or you're unable to gain strength or muscle mass, you may need to increase carbohydrate or protein. If you notice that you gaining unwanted weight or feel physically uncomfortable during training and competition, you may need to lower your carbohydrate or calorie intake. Lean on the foundational principles discussed throughout the first few chapters of this book, and then continue to tweak your fueling plan as you discover what works best for you! The last two chapters will cover some specific considerations and examples that can help all of these things come together.

CHAPTER 12
Special Considerations

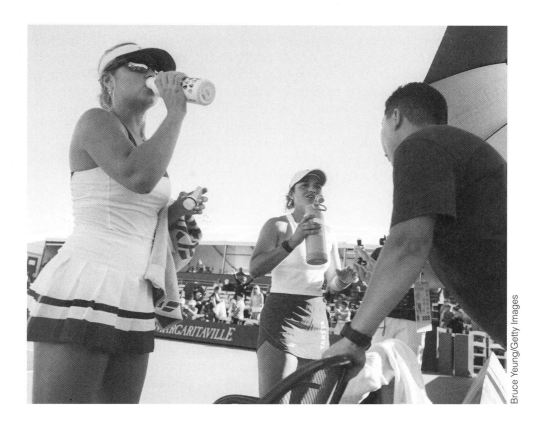

Bruce Yeung/Getty Images

At this point you should have a good understanding of your fueling needs as they pertain to your body size, your activity level, and your training schedule. This should give you a great nutritional base as you work on adding sustainable goals into your routine. However, there are a number of situations that might add different considerations to the plan that you have developed—or even throw a wrench in them completely. This chapter will cover how you can make tweaks to your plan if your sport or position warrants a change in weight, as well as how to manage your energy needs in the event of injury.

Managing Weight Goals

For some athletes, their goals around nutrition may involve gaining or losing weight. It's fair to acknowledge that weight goals can be pertinent to performance, but it's also important to remember that weight and body composition are only one part of performance. Sometimes athletes become overly focused on weight goals and ignore other aspects of performance that may contribute much more to their success, such as sleep, stress management, strength and conditioning, skill development, nutrition, and hydration. If you are adequately addressing those things and still feel that a shift in weight might improve performance, then it is reasonable to work toward a weight goal, but only if you do so safely and appropriately. Losing or gaining weight too quickly or in an unsafe manner is a fast track to derail performance and health.

This chapter will discuss some general tips for promoting safe weight gain and weight loss, but it would also be beneficial for you to work with a dietitian who can take your individual needs and considerations into account, especially if your weight goal involves a large shift in either direction.

Weight Gain

For weight-gain goals, a good rate to aim for is one to two pounds per week. If you are gaining much faster than this, the weight is more likely to come from body fat than muscle. Although you will likely gain some body fat when trying to gain weight, especially when trying to put on an extreme amount of weight, it is ideal for performance to gain more muscle than body fat. You should add 500 to 1,000 calories to your estimated caloric needs (discussed in chapter 1) to help promote weight gain. The following are some general guidelines that can help promote safe weight gain.

Keep Intake High

Support your training with a high-energy (high-calorie) diet. To promote weight gain, your body has to have enough calories on board to promote building muscle and adding mass. Although you'll need more calories, don't forget the basic principles discussed in the first few chapters of this book. You should still aim to have balanced plates with carbohydrate and protein.

When trying to gain weight, athletes often become overly focused on protein. Although adequate protein is necessary to support MPS, it's imperative to not neglect carbohydrate to support training and help meet overall calorie goals. Remember to include foods that are energy dense as well—these have a lot of calories in a small amount of food, so they can help calories add up more quickly without making you feel overly full. Of course, not all energy-dense foods are nutritious, so try to ensure that most of your choices are healthy options. Examples of energy-dense foods that have health benefits include nuts, nut butters, trail mix, olives, olive or canola oil, avocado, guacamole, and cheese.

Certain beverages are also calorie dense and can provide health benefits. These can help add calories to meals and snacks without filling you up as much as food does. Examples of these include milk, chocolate milk, 100 percent fruit or veggie juice, smoothies, and protein shakes.

Be Consistent

Be consistent with your workout and meal plans. Lack of consistency is one of the biggest reasons athletes struggle to meet weight goals. You cannot realistically build muscle without a good strength and conditioning program, so trust your strength coach and work hard in the weight room. Likewise, meeting your calorie goals only a few days a week will not promote weight gain. You don't need to be perfect, but you need meet these goals most days of the week to see true progress, including after reaching your goal weight if you want to keep the weight on.

Remember to eat frequently and consistently—when aiming for high calorie goals, each meal and snack opportunity is key. Skipping meals is one of the quickest ways to derail your goals. Aim to eat a meal or snack (or have a calorie-rich beverage) at least every three to four hours, if not every two to three.

Avoid Quick Fixes

It's not uncommon for athletes who want to gain weight to jump straight to using supplements. Most athletes can meet higher calorie goals and promote weight gain through food alone; however, some supplements marketed toward weight gain like powders, shakes, and bars may be helpful from a convenience standpoint. Creatine can also be helpful in gaining mass if it matches your goals. Remember the discussion in chapter 8 about the risks and seek qualified advice before using supplements. If you are interested in using a supplement, make sure it has undergone third-party testing.

Stay Vigilant

Monitor progress and adjust as needed. As you work toward a weight goal, you will inevitably have ups and downs—weight gain is almost never linear. You may see gains the first few weeks and then plateau. If this happens, evaluate whether you are being consistent with your goals. If you are, you may need to slightly increase your calorie goal to continue to see the same progress.

It is best to only weigh once a week in controlled conditions (same day each week, same time of the day). Weight naturally fluctuates over the course of a day and a week, so weighing more often will not necessarily give you a realistic view of your progress. It's also an easy way to become overly focused on acute changes in body weight. Also avoid weighing right after a workout, when you are likely not fully hydrated and will not get an accurate weight measurement.

Weight Loss

For weight-loss goals, a good rate to aim for is one to two pounds per week. If you are losing weight faster than this, you are likely losing muscle mass, which does not promote performance. Extreme losses can also negatively affect health and be detrimental to bone health and reproductive health. You should subtract 300 to 500 calories from your estimated caloric needs (discussed in chapter 1) to help promote safe weight loss. The following are some general guidelines that can help promote safe weight loss.

Make Those Calories Count

Aim for a nutrient-dense diet. Although you do want to create a caloric deficit to promote weight loss, it's vital that you still provide your body what it needs for health and performance. Don't forget the basic

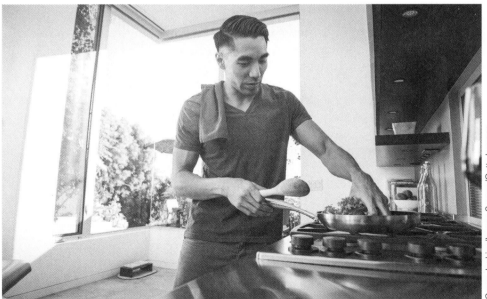

Corey Jenkins/Image Source/Getty Images

Take an individualized approach to weight goals and make sure that your plan is sustainable for the long term.

principles discussed in the first few chapters of this book. You should still aim to have balanced plates with carbohydrate and protein, but strive to add plenty of fruits and vegetables, which don't add up as quickly and can help keep you feeling full.

Limit energy-dense foods and beverages. Your diet doesn't need to be perfect to promote weight loss, but you should aim to choose lean choices often. When it comes to protein choices, try to choose grilled or baked options and limit fried and highly processed options. Try to limit high-fat foods that can add up quickly calorically and leave you unsatisfied, such as bacon, sausage, ribs, wings, pepperoni, fried foods, cheesy or creamy sauces, butter, cookies, cakes, and biscuits. Although you can include drinks you enjoy as part of a weight-loss plan, drinks tend to not be as filling as food and may make it hard to meet calorie goals. Limit choices like soda, sweet tea, high-fat coffee drinks, and alcohol.

Be Consistent

Be consistent with your workout plan. Being active in the weight room will help preserve muscle mass, and an overall higher energy expenditure will help promote weight loss. With this said, ensure that you are not overexercising, which can cause health concerns as well. Stick with the plan outlined by your coaches, and if you are approved to add additional exercise make sure that it is low impact (not hard on your joints).

You should also continue to eat frequently. Just because you have a goal of losing weight doesn't mean that you should skip meals or that you should be hungry. In fact, skipping meals can promote muscle breakdown, which is detrimental to performance. Additionally, skipping meals naturally leaves you feeling hungry, which can lead to intense cravings and potentially to overeating, making it hard to stick to the plan. Cravings like these are often perceived as a lack of willpower, but these are simply a physiological need displayed by your body.

Again, the goal is not to have a perfect diet—such a thing is unattainable and not very enjoyable. A good weight-loss plan can still allow foods you enjoy and flexibility for situations like family dinners, eating out with friends, and parties. You should simply try to follow these guidelines most days of the week; otherwise, you will likely find that you do not meet your goals.

Avoid Quick Fixes

It's not uncommon for athletes who want to lose weight to jump straight to using supplements. However, most supplements marketed toward weight loss don't work—and if they do, you should be concerned as to why. Often they have diuretics or other ingredients that can cause drug-testing concerns as well as be dangerous for your health. Seek qualified advice before using weight-loss supplements.

Stay Vigilant

Monitor progress and adjust as needed. As you work toward a weight goal, you will inevitably have ups and downs—weight loss is almost never linear. You may lose a few pounds quickly at first and then plateau. If this

Energy Availability

Remember, when it comes to weight loss, more is not necessarily better. Keep close tabs on how you're feeling and performing. You might also consider evaluating energy availability, which is defined as energy obtained through nutrition minus energy expended during exercise. If energy availability becomes too low, there is no longer adequate nutrition left for your organs and vital bodily processes, and health can be affected. Energy availability can be calculated by using the following equation:

Energy availability = (daily calorie intake – daily calorie expenditure from exercise) / kg fat free mass (FFM)

If energy availability drops below 30 kilocalories per kilogram FFM, this is a red flag that calorie intake is too low and should be adjusted (see figure 12.1). The ideal energy availability is 45 kilocalories or more per kilogram FFM.

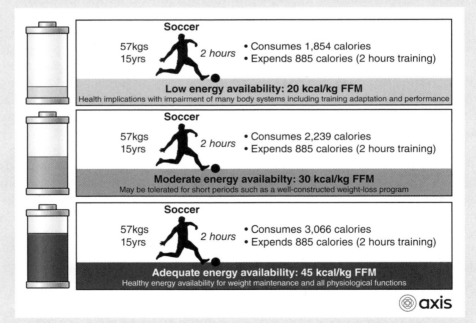

FIGURE 12.1 Energy availability thresholds can help delineate whether or not athletes are meeting their needs.

Adapted by permission from D. Baker, "What is Low Energy Availability and How Do We Calculate It?" Axis Sports Medicine, last modified November 20, 2020, https://www.axissportsmedicine.co.nz/blog/what-is-low-energy-availability-and-how-do-we-calculate-it.

happens, evaluate whether you are being consistent with your goals. If you are, you may need to slightly increase your expenditure or decrease intake to see the same progress.

It is best to only weigh once a week in controlled conditions (same day each week, same time of the day). Weight naturally fluctuates over the course of a day and a week, so weighing more often will not necessarily give you a realistic view of your progress. It's also an easy way to become overly focused on acute changes in body weight.

Injury Recovery

Although something that no athlete wants to deal with, it's nearly inevitable that at one point or another you will have to deal with at least a minor injury. It's important to note that although no amount of good nutrition can take away all risk, solid nutrition habits can help reduce your risk for many modes of injury (especially soft-tissue and bone injuries) and also support a healthy immune system. However, even athletes with the best nutrition habits can still get injured, so the following section will discuss the vital role that nutrition plays in injury recovery.

Supporting Energy Needs Through Recovery

One of the most important factors in recovering from an injury is continuing to adequately support your caloric needs. A common mistake for injured athletes is to assume that because they're not practicing or training their energy expenditure is vastly lower. Although calorie needs may be lower while not training, it's usually not nearly to the extent that one might assume—and if recovering from a significant or traumatic injury it's possible that needs might actually be remain similar. This is because healing takes a considerable number of calories: As noted by Smith-Ryan and colleagues (2020), during injury recovery an athlete's BMR increases to match the energy demands of rebuilding and repairing the damaged tissue.

In addition to factoring in physical activity to determine caloric needs, as discussed in chapter 2 (e.g., using crutches), you should also factor in stress, depending on the type of injury sustained (e.g., postsurgery wound healing). You would multiply your BMR with both the activity factor and this stress factor to calculate your total needs to support healing. Figure 12.2 expands on how you might calculate those needs.

If your estimated expenditure is indeed lower than usual, a simple approach to accommodating this change in calorie needs is to think back to the balanced plates discussed in chapter 2 and aim to have your plate filled with one-half fruits and veggies, one-fourth carbohydrate, and one-fourth protein. This will ensure you get adequate carbohydrate

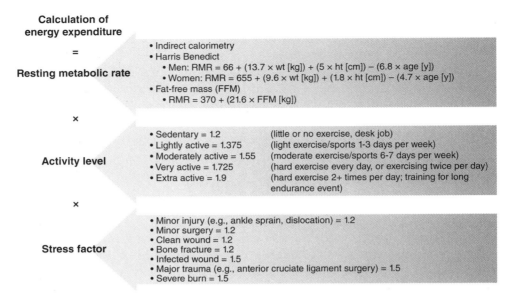

Calculation of energy expenditure

=

Resting metabolic rate

- Indirect calorimetry
- Harris Benedict
  - Men: RMR = 66 + (13.7 × wt [kg]) + (5 × ht [cm]) − (6.8 × age [y])
  - Women: RMR = 655 + (9.6 × wt [kg]) + (1.8 × ht [cm]) − (4.7 × age [y])
- Fat-free mass (FFM)
  - RMR = 370 + (21.6 × FFM [kg])

×

Activity level

- Sedentary = 1.2   (little or no exercise, desk job)
- Lightly active = 1.375   (light exercise/sports 1-3 days per week)
- Moderately active = 1.55 (moderate exercise/sports 6-7 days per week)
- Very active = 1.725   (hard exercise every day, or exercising twice per day)
- Extra active = 1.9   (hard exercise 2+ times per day; training for long endurance event)

×

Stress factor

- Minor injury (e.g., ankle sprain, dislocation) = 1.2
- Minor surgery = 1.2
- Clean wound = 1.2
- Bone fracture = 1.2
- Infected wound = 1.5
- Major trauma (e.g., anterior cruciate ligament surgery) = 1.5
- Severe burn = 1.5

FIGURE 12.2   Athletes can account for additional energy needs while recovering from injuries by multiplying their resting metabolic rate with their activity level and stress factor from that injury.

Reprinted by permission from A.E. Smith-Ryan, K.R. Kirsch, H.E. Saylor et al., "Nutritional Considerations and Strategies to Facilitate Injury Recovery and Rehabilitation," *Journal of Athletic Training* 55, no. 9 (2020): 918-930, https://doi:10.4085/1062-6050-550-19.

and protein to support recovery and healing but help keep overall caloric intake balanced while you're unable to exercise as much.

You should also plan to continue eating frequently while recovering from an injury. It can be easy to let this habit lapse if you find your appetite is lower while not as physically active, but remember that one of the benefits of eating frequently is helping promote MPS. So though it's reasonable to adjust portion sizes and perhaps cut out some snacking while injured, you should still strive to eat regularly and avoid skipping meals to help prevent unnecessary muscle loss. Although it may not be realistic to eliminate them completely, you might also try to limit foods high in unhealthy fats and refined sugar while you're injured, as well as beverages such as soda and alcohol. This is in part because of the excess calories that these foods can contribute while expenditure is lower, but also because these foods can contribute to inflammatory responses, which are already heightened during injury recovery.

It is well supported that protein needs are higher during recovery from injury. Tipton (2015) suggests that during the rehabilitation process, athletes should strive for protein intakes of at least 1.6 grams per kilogram per day and ideally closer to 2.0 to 3.0 grams per kilogram per day. He also emphasizes including leucine-rich foods (3 g per serving), because leucine is the primary amino acid responsible for stimulating MPS. One primary reason for these higher protein needs is to prevent MPB. It is nearly impossible to avoid muscle atrophy completely during injury recovery, especially if you have limited mobility or an immobilized limb. However, adequate protein intake can help attenuate this loss and set you up for an easier return to training when you're recovered.

In addition to appropriate overall calorie and protein intake, good hydration habits are essential to recovery. It can be easy to let hydration fall to the wayside when recovering from an injury because you are not working out and replacing sweat losses nearly as much as usual, but adequate water intake is key in many healing processes. Although these overall practices are good for any injury, there are also some considerations and specific nutrients that are helpful in recovering from different kinds of injuries.

Soft-Tissue Injuries

Soft-tissue injuries include muscle strains and pulls as well as injuries to a joint or ligament. Often these injuries are related to reduced pliability of muscles, lack of flexibility, or sometimes uneven strength between synergistic muscle groups. In addition to the general recommendations discussed previously, one nutritional intervention that has gained popularity in the realm of rehabbing soft-tissue injuries is using collagen and vitamin C. Collagen is the most prevalent protein in connective tissue, and vitamin C is crucial in the process of synthesizing collagen. Research by Shaw and colleagues (2017) suggests that adding vitamin C–rich gelatin (a collagen-rich food) to an intermittent exercise program improves collagen synthesis and could play a beneficial role in injury prevention and tissue repair. Although the research on collagen and vitamin C for collagen synthesis is mixed, a study by Lis and Baar (2019) found that vitamin C–enriched gelatin supplementation may improve collagen synthesis when taken one hour prior to exercise; procollagen levels tended to increase by about 20 percent compared to baseline.

If you are recovering from a soft-tissue injury and interested in using collagen as part of your rehabilitation plan, it is suggested to consume 15 grams of collagen with 50 milligrams of vitamin C about 30 to 60 minutes prior to starting rehabilitation work. These could be consumed as separate products or in one combined product, the latter of which has become more popular. Regardless of which you choose, remember the considerations for choosing a safe supplement discussed in chapter 8.

In lieu of a supplement you could also eat foods rich in gelatin, one of the most common being Jell-O. Although the exact amount would depend on the brand and the preparation, a general estimate is that you would need to eat about 1 cup of Jell-O to get 15 grams of collagen. If

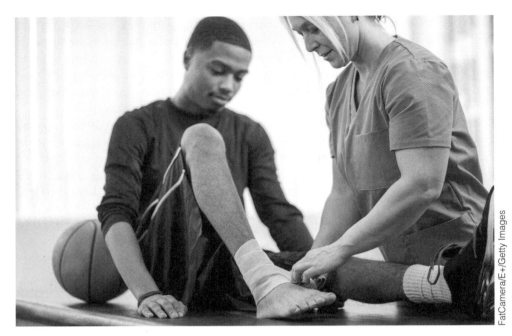

FatCamera/E+/Getty Images

Make sure to include collagen in your diet to aid in the repair and strengthening of soft tissues after an injury.

you do decide to use Jell-O, don't forget the vitamin C component. You could prepare the gelatin using vitamin C–rich juice (e.g., orange juice, apple juice) rather than water, or you could eat the Jell-O with a side of vitamin C–rich fruit to get the desired synergistic effect.

Bone Injuries

Bone injuries include stress fractures, contusions, and fractures to any bone. It is well known that nutrition plays an important role in bone health—specifically, adequate amount of calcium and vitamin D are crucial to support the body's ability to build bone in childhood and adolescence and to prevent breakdown of bone in adulthood. Although those nutrients are the key players, vitamin K, magnesium, and phosphorous are also important. Bone health is not generally something that can be acutely affected, but rather is a result of nutrition and training habits over many years. It's crucial for young athletes (and parents of young athletes) to understand that humans are only able to build bone into their early to mid-20s. After that point, we only lose bone. It's therefore vital to maximize bone building in those early years and not put yourself at risk for not only bone injury, but also low bone mineral density and related issues such as osteopenia and osteoporosis later in life.

Underfueling is one of the main causes of poor bone health in childhood and adolescence. This is partly a result of lack of adequate nutrients, but also because underfueling negatively affects hormone levels that help promote bone building—the same hormones that support healthy menstruation in girls and women—which is why poor bone health and amenorrhea are often seen simultaneously. Although long-term habits are key, in the instance of bone injury, there are some nutrition interventions that can help promote healing.

If you have a stress fracture or compound fracture, you should consider using a third-party tested calcium and vitamin D supplement while healing. Although you should always prioritize your doctor's recommendations, a common dosage when healing from a bone injury would be 600 milligrams of calcium and 1,000 to 2,000 IU of vitamin D daily. It's possible that your doctor would want to test your vitamin D levels, and in the event your vitamin D was low, they would likely increase the amount to upward of 5,000 to 10,000 IU per day.

Although a supplement is a surefire way to get vitamin D levels up, there are also many foods rich in vitamin D, such as milk, cheese, yogurt, fish, and fortified orange juice and cereals. As discussed in chapter 6, vitamin D is fat soluble, so it's important to consume some dietary fat to promote absorption.

Concussion

Concussion is a mild traumatic brain injury caused by a blow to the head that results in cognitive symptoms such as headache, confusion, lack of coordination, nausea, vomiting, memory loss, and fatigue. No two concussions are the same, and severity of symptoms and time to recovery tends to vary wildly between individuals. Nutritional interventions for treatment of concussions are still relatively new, but increased energy needs when recovering from a concussion are widely accepted (figure 12.3). Despite lower expenditure while resting and recovering from a concussion, it's imperative to not underfuel and impede the brain's recovery.

When it comes to supplementation, omega-3 fatty acids generally lead the way. Barrett, McBurney, and Ciappio (2014) found a dose of 40 milligrams per kilogram per day immediately after injury to be effective in adults. Although supplementing omega-3 fatty acids after a concussion is advisable, there is also research to support that consistent use of omega-3 fatty acids prior to head injury can have neuroprotective effects (Mishra et al. 2022; Oliver, Anzalone, and Turner 2018). With this in mind, athletes who participate in sports that make them prone to concussions (such as football, soccer, or wrestling) might consider taking a low dose of 1 to 2 grams of an omega-3 fatty acid supplement; this is discussed further

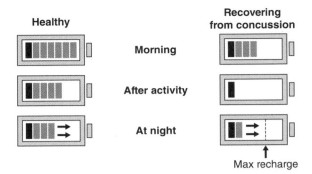

FIGURE 12.3   The brain's ability to recharge its energy reserves are markedly reduced after suffering a concussion.

Reprinted by permission from E. Morales-Grahl, "What Happens to Your Brain When You Get a Concussion: A Deeper Dive," Concussion Alliance, accessed September 25, 2023, www.concussionalliance.org/what-happens-to -your-brain-a-deeper-dive.

in chapter 8. Curcumin has also piqued some interest, and work by Zhu and colleagues (2014) and Wu, Ying, and Gomez-Pinilla (2006) highlight its potential to reduce tissue damage and improve cognition after concussive brain injuries. The accepted dose for curcumin is 100 milligrams per kilogram containing 95 percent curcuminoids.

Creatine is also an exciting nutritional intervention for concussion treatment. As noted by Smith-Ryan and colleagues (2020), creatine in the brain is reduced after suffering a brain injury. Creatine supplementation may therefore balance out ATP and reduce negative side effects on energy status. Recommended dosages vary considerably—anywhere from 4 to 20 grams per day. One study by Ainsley Dean and colleagues (2017) found that a larger dose of 0.4 grams per kilogram per day for six months after a concussion improved cognitive function and decreased headaches, dizziness, and fatigue in children. As Smith-Ryan and colleagues (2020) point out, creatine is a low-risk approach that shows a lot of promise. As outlined in chapter 8, taking 20 grams per day of a third-party tested creatine monohydrate product is a good general guideline. Rather than taking a full dose all at once, you can divide the 20-gram amount into four smaller doses of 5g each throughout the day.

Postsurgical Care

In some cases, an injury might also involve surgery to repair the injured bone, ligament, or tendon. When this is the case, all of the previously mentioned strategies still apply. However, the demand for amino acids specifically would be expected to rise even more to support the healing of incisions, tissue grafts, and other secondary trauma sustained during surgery (Smith-Ryan et al. 2020). Increased protein intake in the days before surgery may help minimize muscle loss and accelerate recovery. Hirsch, Wolfe, and Ferrando (2021) note that standard protein requirements of at least 1.6 grams per kilogram per day must be met during this time frame, though recommendations can range as high as 2 to 3 grams per kilogram per day.

Additionally, there are some micronutrients that are especially helpful in promoting wound healing. The amino acids arginine and glutamine; vitamins A, B, C, and D; zinc; and iron are all essential for the inflammatory process and the synthesis of collagen, which are crucial in promoting the creation of new tissue as the wound heals (Barchitta et al. 2019). Because arginine and glutamine aren't commonly found in a multivitamin with these other nutrients, individual supplements are recommended in doses between 6 and 10 grams. Additionally, you could consider a product like Juven, which is designed to combine all of these nutrients with the goal of promoting wound healing. The anti-inflammatory and antioxidant properties of curcumin might also be beneficial for many processes involved in wound healing (Smith Ryan et al. 2020); recommended dosages range from 500 to 2,000 milligrams per day during healing. Eating foods rich in these nutrients is a great step in promoting an efficient road to recovery, as is including a multivitamin that can help ensure you meet your needs. Finally, ensure you have good hygiene practices and follow any wound care instructions provided by your doctors and health care team.

As highlighted in this chapter, there are many situations that warrant taking an individualized approach to your nutrition plan and the timing surrounding it. If you have the unfortunate experience of sustaining an injury while training or competing, it can be easy to let nutrition fall to the wayside, especially considering that injuries (especially significant ones) are usually accompanied by some amount of stress. However, as hard as it might feel to refocus, the best thing you can do for your body and your ability to get back to doing what you love is to prioritize hydration, get enough macro- and micronutrients, and recognize and adjust for any gaps in your diet.

The last chapter will address some additional considerations that can help you plan for different environments and troubleshoot circumstances that affect your schedule and your access to different nutritional resources.

CHAPTER 13
Prep and Plan Ahead

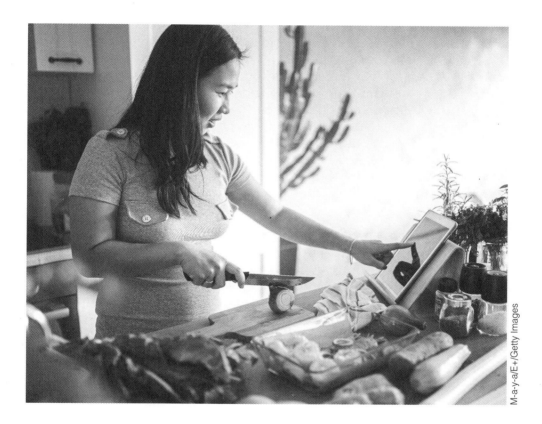

No matter what level of athlete you are, managing a busy schedule is one of the trickiest parts of finding success. Prepping and planning ahead can make a huge difference in your ability to carry out a plan and meet your goals. Taking the time to think through logistics can not only save you time, but also help you stick to a plan and ultimately reduce stress and anxiety. It can also help promote better nutritional goals—lack of planning often leads to outcomes like quickly grabbing fast food or not eating at all. This chapter will address a few of the most common nutrition challenges for high school athletes, college athletes, and athletes working a full-time job.

High School Athletes

High school athletes have many unique challenges, but one of the biggest is that they spend all day in school and are often limited in their ability to get food outside of the school setting. School lunches (and breakfasts) are standardized servings with little flexibility and may not be enough for an athlete with a very high expenditure. Especially if you are a dual-sport athlete with overlapping seasons or playing on both your high school team and a club team, it's important not to underestimate your needs. Multiple practices a day add up, and adequate calories and recovery are important for success and avoiding injuries. Additionally, high school students are often at the mercy of their parents or guardians in terms of what food is available at home. Finally, students are also usually unable to drive until junior or senior year, which limits their ability to be independent with some of these considerations. Although you cannot control everything, planning ahead can help abate some of these problems.

Fueling Before and During School

As discussed early in this book, meal frequency is important for success. Breakfast is too important to skip, so if you are serious about your athletic goals, you will hopefully be willing to trade 5 or 10 minutes of sleep to make sure you have time to eat breakfast. It doesn't need to be fancy and could even just be a bowl of cereal and milk, a smoothie, a microwave breakfast sandwich, or a protein shake or bar. Though simple, all of these ideas have carbohydrate and protein and are significantly better options than not eating at all. You might mention to your parent or guardian that it would be helpful for you to have some of these options available (or other breakfast items that sound good to you). If logistics or resources are a concern, consider taking advantage of your school's free breakfast program. This program can be a lifesaver for many high school students!

Similarly, the importance of lunch should not be underestimated, especially because this is often the last meal before you practice in the afternoon. Most schools have lunch menus available ahead of time, so take a few minutes each week to see if the options are something that you like and will eat. If so, great! If not, plan ahead for what you will do instead. Some schools have ala carte options, which can be good choices if approached purposefully. Remember the balanced plates in chapter 2 and aim to choose something that has carbohydrate, protein, and a fruit or vegetable if possible—just getting French fries from the ala carte line is not setting yourself up for your best performance when practice rolls around that afternoon.

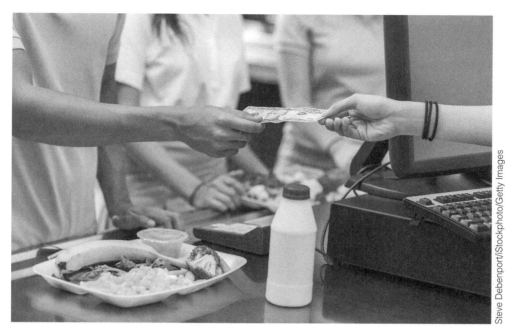

School cafeterias almost always offer healthy options to keep you fueled and focused during the day.

You can also consider packing a lunch. If realistic for you, this can be a fantastic way to ensure that you have appropriate portion sizes and choices you enjoy that support performance. Similarly to breakfast, if this is something you would like to do, make sure you communicate with whoever does the grocery shopping about what you are hoping to have available. Packing a lunch can be as fancy or as simple as you choose. It can be a nice way to repurpose leftovers, especially if you have a way to heat them up at school. If you don't have a way to microwave a meal, you might be better off with options like sandwiches, wraps, or salads—as long as you can get enough calories and carbohydrate in your options. Even a good old fashioned PB&J can be a great fallback if you don't have anything fresh on hand. Regardless of what you choose, remember your balanced plates and try to make sure whatever you choose has carbohydrate, protein, and a fruit or vegetable. Portions should be enough to keep you full the rest of the school day and ensure you'll have fuel on board for practice.

In addition to packing something to eat for lunch, consider packing some extra snacks. A carbohydrate-rich snack before you start practice or training is a great way to make sure you are energized and ready to perform at a high level. This can be something simple like crackers, pretzels, a granola bar, piece of fruit, applesauce, or even a Gatorade. If you struggle with getting enough in at meals or are struggling to keep

TABLE 13.1   **Easy Packed Lunch Options**

Carbohydrate	Protein	Fruits and veggies
Whole-wheat bread	Turkey, cheese	Grapes
Large tortilla	Shredded chicken, cheese	Lettuce, tomato, guacamole
Whole-wheat bread, jelly	Peanut butter, string cheese	Banana, carrot sticks
Pasta salad	Chicken breast, mozzarella cheese	Tomatoes, cucumbers
Crackers, pretzels	Deli meat, cheese, hummus	Olives, cucumbers, carrots
Rice	Steak, cheese	Peppers, onions, salsa

your weight up and keep up with energy expenditure, you might also want to pack some easy-to-eat snacks to have at passing periods or other times during your day. Table 13.1 provides some ideas on how to pack for meals on the go.

Other challenges for high school athletes include the tight passing periods and rules around what you can have with you in class. Some schools prohibit having water bottles or food in class, which can make it challenging to stay hydrated or eat snacks. If your school has these rules, you should make a concerted effort to drink water during passing periods and at lunch so that you are not playing catch-up right before practice.

Fueling Outside of School

For high school athletes, challenges may span beyond the school day. They often have minimal, if any, control over what is being served at home or even what is available. If possible, communicate to a parent or guardian some of the needs you've identified through reading this book. If budget is a concern, you can also reference table 13.2, shown later.

Eating out may also be a regular part of your routine depending on practice times and the commute between school, practice, and home. Although it may not be quite as nutritious as eating a home cooked meal, it is an inevitable part of many athletes' schedules, so it's best to approach it in a purposeful manner so as to avoid eating something too heavy just before practice, or missing out on key nutrients during critical time frames.

Another often unavoidable challenge for high school athletes is the late nights that sometimes come from trying to catch up on studying (or possibly their social life). Many people assume that eating late at night is automatically a bad thing and will ignore their hunger cues after a certain time. However, as long as your choice is a purposeful one, it's actually a great idea to have a late night snack. Remember the recommendation that you should try to eat frequently, every three to four hours—if you ate dinner around 6 or 7 p.m. and it is now midnight, it would be wise to have a snack. The approach should be the same as any other time; look to combine carbohydrate and protein. Some simple examples would include cereal and milk, yogurt with fruit or granola, popcorn and beef jerky, crackers and cheese, or a PB&J and milk.

Overall, spend a little time up front looking at your schedule and thinking through what you might need to do to make your nutrition plan a success. Make sure you communicate with parents or guardians so that they can help you, and make sure you use resources available to you, especially if budget is limited!

College Athletes

For many college athletes, this time in their lives proves to be a strange mix of newfound independence and highly structured environment. Although the specifics depend on the institution and the level of play, most college athletes have a jam-packed schedule and an entire team of professionals dedicated to their success—it is not uncommon to have access to a strength coach, athletic trainer, team physician, dietitian, psychologist, academic advisors, and tutors, just to name a few. In addition to people, you will likely have access to other resources, including some number of meals and snacks, depending on your institution and the season. This is an incredible benefit that helps ensure that you're getting adequate food to fuel your training. However, it can also lend itself to overreliance, leaving you unable to fend for yourself when it comes to grocery shopping and cooking.

With all this in mind, there are many ways college athletes can maximize their experience. First and foremost, take full advantage these resources. Get to know the team and trust their expertise. As an athlete you may be targeted by people trying to convince you to use a certain product or eat or train a certain way, but I encourage you to rely on the team at your institution—they are paid to understand and care for you, not sell you supplements or workout and meal plans. In a day and age when social media pumps out misinformation by the second, you are lucky to have a dedicated team of individuals who went to school for their specific areas of study and can provide you nonbiased information to meet your unique needs. Along the same lines, if you are provided with a meal plan or access to team meals and snacks, use them! One of the most frustrating things I hear from college athletes is that they aren't using their meal plan or that they skip team meals. Even if you don't love the options on a particular day, try to find something suitable for before and after training. Even if you don't eat a full meal, by getting in some fuel and hydrating, you are taking a small step toward improving your performance.

Dorm Life

Dining halls, specifically, are often challenging for college athletes. The options may be limited, and even items that you generally enjoy might not be prepared the way you're used to. Although there's not a lot you can do about the menu or preparation methods, there are some tips that can help you navigate these spaces so that you don't waste an important (and pricey) resource like a meal plan!

- *Check before you go.* If possible, check the menu ahead of time. Although the facility closest to your apartment or dorm may be the most convenient, it may not have what you prefer. Many universities have multiple dining facilities that have different menus available on a website or app. By checking ahead, you can choose the menu that sounds the best and give yourself the best chance of properly fueling. These are also particularly helpful if you have allergies, intolerances, or other dietary restrictions.

- *Take a lap.* When you get there, make a lap. It can be easy to gravitate to the first thing you see when you walk in the door or to just put food on your plate as you see it, but take a minute or two to make a lap and see all the options. Not only will this make you more likely to find items you enjoy, but you will also be more likely to build a balanced plate, as discussed in chapter 2.

- *Take another lap.* If you make a lap and don't see anything you like, don't immediately assume there's nothing there for you. Consider having some go-to staples on days that you don't see any hot items that sound good.

- *Get creative.* For proteins, consider making a deli sandwich or grabbing yogurt or cottage cheese from the salad bar. Add protein-rich toppings to a salad, like hard-boiled eggs, turkey, ham, chickpeas, or black beans. For carbohydrates, make a PB&J or have a bowl of cereal. Get a bowl of fruit or applesauce from the salad bar. Have a roll or breadstick.

- *Fill your plate.* People tend to eat fewer fruits and vegetables at dining halls than they otherwise would. Make an effort to always grab each component of a performance plate (carbs, protein, and fruits and veggies), especially if they have options that you like. Utilize the salad bar. Even grabbing something simple like a banana, applesauce or canned fruit, a small glass of fruit juice, or a smoothie is a great way to get some fruits and veggies in.

- *Hydrate.* With many different options available, make it a point to have at least one glass of fluid while you sit and eat. Sticking to options like water, tea, and milk over soda can be helpful from an overall hydration standpoint.

- *Don't skip dessert.* For some, having access to dessert options all the time in a dining hall can make it challenging to use moderation around those items. Remember, you do not need to avoid these foods completely. In fact, when people try to avoid a craving it usually makes them want it more and feel more out of control when they do have it. If you find that it's hard for you to control your portion sizes when eating in the dining hall, consider taking your dessert to go. By grabbing a cookie or an ice cream cone on your way out the door, you will be able to enjoy those foods without feeling pressured by the urge to go back up for seconds and thirds!

- *Grab a friend.* Enjoy fellowship with your friends and teammates! Dining hall settings are an interesting environment and often full of many different people—don't overlook how fun connecting over a meal can be. While you're enjoying that company, however, keep your eyes on your own plate. What your teammates are eating is none of your business, and everyone has unique likes, dislikes, and nutritional needs. Commenting on someone else's plate isn't helpful and can lead to unhealthy behaviors for yourself and your teammates. If you have a concern about a teammate's behaviors around food, mention it to a staff member—ideally one within sports medicine or nutrition.

Off-Campus

Dining hall meal plans and team meals are a fantastic resource—but as mentioned, they can make it easy to get by without learning your way around a kitchen. A time will come when you will need to fend for yourself, and you don't want to become reliant on takeout or frozen dinners, both of which can be expensive and are not usually the healthiest approach. You are therefore encouraged to spend some time now learning how to do basic things in the kitchen—in part because there will certainly be times during the year when team meals are not available, but also because college is a time when most people are learning these skills.

Learn how to boil water, how to cook chicken and ground beef, and how to make eggs. Understand basic concepts of food safety—for example, never use the same cutting board for both raw meat and vegetables. Learn how to use a Crock-Pot or an air fryer. If you want simple, easy recipes, google "simple easy recipes." If you don't know how to do something, watch a YouTube tutorial. Thanks to the Internet, there is no reason to not have basic proficiency in the kitchen.

Changing Schedules

Another common challenge of college life is simply the busy schedule. You'll be asked to juggle a lot: classes, practice, conditioning, film sessions, and travel. You may also have to squeeze in rehabbing an injury, going to extra tutors, and possibly even a job, depending on your financial situation. And don't forget about a social life! It's easy to see why it quickly becomes hard to figure out how to work meals and sleep into the equation. I would advise you to sit down with your schedule each semester (or any other time that your schedule makes a dramatic shift) and ask yourself, "when am I going to eat?" Sometimes you may have natural breaks in your schedule that will make it easy to run home and make something or stop by a local restaurant and grab a quick meal. However, other times you may quickly notice that there's not much time at all. With this information, plan ahead! If you need to pack something, make sure you do. Even something simple like a PB&J, protein bar or shake, and some fruit can make an easy lunch that doesn't need refrigeration and can have you fueled up for practice later that day. Remember, going too long without eating sets you up for low energy stores, muscle loss, and ultimately decreased performance. Also make sure you always bring a water bottle with you—as discussed in chapter 7, you can't show up to practice, start drinking water, and expect to be fully hydrated. If you have trouble remembering to actually take drinks while you're in class or running around campus, consider setting reminders on your phone or using a hydration-tracking app that can prompt you to hit hydration goals.

All of these things can be even more challenging during especially busy time frames like final exams, project deadlines, or competitive seasons. Although difficult, staying on top of your nutrition plan during these times can be even more important to elicit the desired performance in both sport and the classroom. Time management tends to be crucial— both for scheduling enough time for what needs to get done, but also making sure that you schedule time to eat! You might consider planning to study at a quiet local café or restaurant or packing snacks that you can munch on while you study or travel.

Travel

Although not completely unique to college sports, travel is certainly a big challenge for college athletes, especially when a trip spans many days and multiple time zones. Of course, many aspects of team travel are not within your control, including travel times, accommodations, and most meals. However, it is standard practice at most levels to provide meals on the road, so ensure you take advantage of those and try to have the same balanced plates that you would have at home. Sometimes eating at restaurants can make it hard to have a balanced plate, because you are more likely to gravitate toward fun foods—especially when someone else is footing the bill! Although you can certainly enjoy some fun foods on the road, remember that you're there for a reason: to compete in your sport. Try to limit high-fat foods the closer you get to game day. For more on precompetition fueling, see chapters 10 and 11.

Hydration is also important while traveling—especially when you are flying. The low humidity of airplane cabin air coupled with the altitude causes increased fluid loss via respiration and can lead to dehydration. Make sure you drink frequently to stay hydrated and consider including an electrolyte supplement or beverage while flying. It can also help to pack snacks for airplane travel given that turnaround can be tight and most flights no longer offer substantial snacks or meals. Consider packing some granola or protein bars, nuts or trail mix, jerky, or even fruit.

Although these suggestions are specific to airplane travel, many of the same principles apply to car or bus travel, especially over long distances. It's important to pack snacks and potentially even light meals, as well as plenty of fluids. When not limited by an airline's rules, you can also get creative: Pack a small cooler with options like sandwiches, yogurt, string cheese, hard boiled eggs, and more. With any travel, your goal for eating

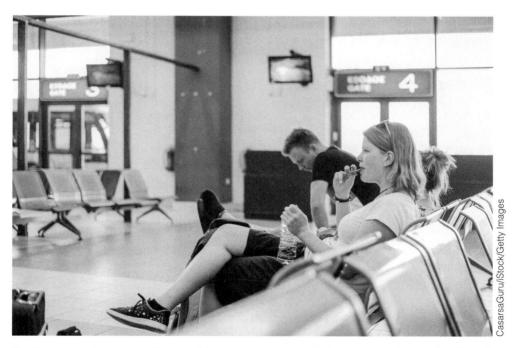

Don't rely on airport vending machines or restaurants to keep you fueled during travel. Bring along healthy snacks for long stopovers and delays when you fly.

frequency and timing should remain the same as usual—eat every three to four hours to maintain energy levels and promote muscle synthesis.

Working 9 to 5

You may have thought you were busy as a student—and then you got out in the real world and realized you had it pretty good in college! There's no doubt that working full time is a whole different kind of grind that poses all kinds of new, unique challenges for those still training at a high level.

One of the biggest challenges is simply the time you must dedicate to full-time work. Long gone are the days when you built your schedule around your workouts or practices. Now the trick becomes squeezing your workouts into that busy schedule. If you take your training and fitness seriously, you'll need to spend some time really assessing your schedule to figure out when you can get your workout in, which will dictate other aspects of your schedule, like meals and snacks. For some, it may mean getting up early and getting your training in before you go to work, whereas others may not be able to get it in until afterward. Depending on your place of work and its access or proximity to a gym, you may even be able to work out over a lunch break or another chunk of time during the day. Whatever works for you, stick to the plan and ensure that you can still get meals in around the rest of your schedule. It's important that you still eat every three to four hours, and with a full-time job that will likely take some additional planning.

Planning Your Meals

To start, ensure you eat breakfast, even if it's something quick and on the go. As discussed in earlier chapters, it's imperative that you eat frequently to support performance, promote MPS, and prevent MPB. If you are doing your training in the morning before work, have something small and carb-rich before the workout (reference chapter 3 for some great carb-rich snacks). Your postworkout snack and breakfast can likely be one and the same; this doesn't need to be anything complicated. Cereal and milk, overnight oats, and eggs and toast are all simple examples of carb and protein combos that could fulfill postworkout needs. Of course, portions should be adjusted to individual needs, and you can consider adding toppings like cheese, avocado, or condiments as well as drinks like milk or juice if you need to boost calories. If time is a concern, you may even brainstorm something you could eat in the car, like a smoothie, breakfast burrito, or breakfast sandwich—especially if you have a long commute. Again, this can be complemented by juice, milk, or a protein shake if you need a calorie boost.

For some working athletes the most challenging meal is lunch. I highly recommend you consider packing a lunch, especially if your office is limited in terms of nearby food options. Because the average lunch out costs around $10, going out for lunch most days of the week would cost you almost $200 per month on lunch alone. By spending 5 to 10 minutes at the end of the night prepping a lunch for the next day, you can not only save money but ensure that you have a nutritious meal waiting for you that adequately supports your training needs.

Lunch may be an excellent time to use leftovers or prep something easy like a sandwich, wrap, soup, or bowl. This meal should be treated like any other and balanced with carbs, protein, and a fruit or vegetable if possible. In addition to bringing lunch, it's great to pack some protein-rich snacks as well as some fruit or vegetables to snack on while you're at work. Not only can this help prevent hunger, but it can also help you ramp up your consumption of these foods. If you struggle to include enough fruit or veggies, having them available at work—where you are more or less stuck with them—increases the chances of snacking on those foods compared to when you're at home and may more easily choose something else. If you have snacks on hand, you're also less likely to gravitate toward vending machine snacks or the office treats that often get brought in, which tend to have lower nutritional content.

Prep Ahead

In general, meal prepping can be helpful for busy schedules, but people often make it more complicated than necessary. The image that social media portrays of meal prepping is one that involves 50 different containers spread out on the counter and a full day of measuring, cooking, and portioning out ingredients. However, the reality can be much simpler and less daunting. The first step toward simple meal prep is ensuring you have groceries at home. You're more likely to stick to your plan when you have everything on hand that you need. If budget is a concern, see table 13.2 for a list of budget-friendly performance foods.

The following tips can also help you save money at the grocery store:

- Plan your meals for the week
- Buying fresh fruits and veggies in-season and on sale
- Buy frozen fruits and veggies in bulk
- Buy protein on sale in bulk and freeze extras
- Buy the store brand instead of name brand
- Use your store's rewards program
- Use coupons

TABLE 13.2   **Right Food, Right Price: Cheap and Nutritious Foods for Fueling on a Budget**

Cost-effective carb-rich foods	Cost-effective protein-rich foods	Cost-effective fruits and veggies
Rice	Frozen chicken breasts	Bananas
Pasta	Frozen tilapia or salmon	Apples
Bread	Canned chicken	Oranges
Tortillas	Canned tuna or salmon	Pears
Oatmeal	Eggs	Cucumbers
Grits	Beans	Baby carrots
Potatoes	Lentils	Celery
Beans	Milk	Broccoli
Lentils	Yogurt	Frozen fruit
	Cottage cheese	Frozen veggies

Before you go grocery shopping, make a list. Not only will this help ensure you leave the store with what you came for, but also prevent you from leaving with a bunch of stuff you didn't need. When you go about making your grocery list, start by thinking through each meal. What will you eat for breakfast, lunch, and dinner that week? For dinner especially, brainstorm a couple different dishes you can make. They don't have to be complicated or include a bunch of different ingredients. It could be as simple as deciding you're going to make tacos and pasta that week. Get ingredients to make those dishes, and make enough to have leftovers if possible. In doing so you've ensured that you have multiple meals covered, whether you choose to use those leftovers for another dinner or bring them in your lunch the next day.

If you're thinking "I don't even know where to start," there are lots of great ways to gather some inspiration. You might start by looking for some accounts on social media that share recipes (search "quick recipes" or "easy meals" on Instagram, TikTok, or Pinterest). You could also purchase a cookbook or two that are centered around simple meals, minimal cleanup, or meal prepping. It's also worth asking friends or family members who enjoy cooking for a couple of their favorite recipes to get you started!

In addition to getting the ingredients for the meals you have planned, it's also helpful to have simple (and shelf-stable) options available at home, especially if you frequently train late or lack motivation after getting home from work. Have frozen protein options that you can throw in the oven like chicken breasts or meatballs, or microwave beans and add them to salads or bowls. Buy rice or pasta packets that you can microwave in a minute or two, or pop a potato in the microwave for six to eight minutes for a baked potato. Have frozen steamable veggie packets or canned vegetables and fruit. Although you don't want to rely on frozen and microwaveable options 100 percent of the time, they can absolutely play a role in your nutrition plan, and their convenience increases the chance that you'll stick to your plan and not get takeout or skip a meal completely.

One option for those who aren't super comfortable in the kitchen are meal subscription services, of which there are many. Although using one of these services will almost always cost more than buying and preparing food on your own, it does have the potential to save you a significant amount of time, so weighing those factors is important as you consider if this might be a good approach for you. If you decide that the cost is worth it for you, look at the meals the subscription has available and evaluate whether they meet some of the goals that you've developed from the earlier chapters of this book: Are the meals balanced with carbohydrate, protein, and fruit and vegetables? Are the portion sizes appropriate for your needs? If they fit those criteria, look into whether they have the option to sample some meals. Many of these services routinely send out coupons or promote trial periods. This can be a nice way to find out if the meals seem like foods you would enjoy.

Although all very different situations, many of the common challenges for athletes remain the same. Your time is stretched thin, and many aspects of your schedule, meals, and activities are out of your control. With this in mind, controlling the things you can control is a must. By planning for the unique challenges posed by your sport and your life, you can set yourself up for success.

Whew—you made it! You've learned a lot about the difference sports nutrition and nutrient timing can make on so many aspects of your performance. You've learned how to determine your specific needs as an athlete and how to apply them to real-life situations. You also have some tools in hand to help you conquer the many challenges that will inevitably present themselves on your athletic journey, and I hope that you're feeling inspired to create some goals.

As my last piece of advice I'll leave you with this: Even the best sports nutrition plan isn't perfect, and it isn't permanent. Life happens, and a good nutrition plan should allow some room for it. Make sure your plan allows you to enjoy the vacation with your family, to join your friends for a drink or a coffee, and to have a fun treat with your child on your way home from the game. As you progress through your career, your training may change, your lifestyle may change as you have a family or change jobs, you may battle injuries, and you'll eventually face retirement. All of these different seasons of life require some adjustments, but they should all be built on the same foundational principles that you're leaning on today. Best of luck, and happy fueling!

Appendix

Throughout the chapters we followed three athletes and highlighted their various needs. Now we'll break down just how we calculated those needs. As a reminder:

Athlete 1: Jenny

Jenny is 22 years old. She is 5 feet, 6 inches (167.64 cm) tall and weighs 140 pounds (63.50 kg). She is a competitive soccer player playing at the collegiate level.

Athlete 2: Doug

Doug is 45 years old. He is 5 feet, 10 inches (177.8 cm) tall and weighs 165 pounds (74.84 kg). He is an endurance athlete who regularly trains for and participates in marathons and triathlons.

Athlete 3: Thomas

Thomas is 18 years old. He is 6 feet, 4 inches (193.04 cm) tall and weighs 285 pounds (129.27 kg). He is an American football player competing at the collegiate level with hopes of playing professionally.

Chapter 2

We calculated each athlete's total energy needs using the Mifflin-St. Jeor equation.

Jenny

For Jenny, we start by converting any values needed:

CONVERT WEIGHT FROM POUNDS TO KILOGRAMS

weight in pounds / 2.205 = weight in kg

Weight in lbs	Equation	Weight in kg
140	140 / 2.205	63.50 kg

CONVERT HEIGHT FROM FEET AND INCHES TO CENTIMETERS

(feet × 12 + inches) × 2.54 = height in cm

Height in feet and inches	Equation	Height in cm
5 ft 6 in	(5 × 12 + 6) × 2.54	167.64 cm

Next, we plug the values into:

MIFFLIN-ST. JEOR EQUATION FOR BMR FOR WOMEN

BMR (kcal/day) = (10 × weight in kg) + (6.25 × height in cm) − (5 × age in years) − 161
BMR = (10 × 63.50) + (6.25 × 167.64) − (5 × 22) − 161
BMR = 635 + 1047.75 − 110 − 161
BMR = 1411.75 kcal/day

Therefore, the estimated BMR for Jenny would be approximately 1,412 kilocalories per day using the Mifflin-St. Jeor equation.

Doug

For Doug, we follow the same steps to start.

CONVERT WEIGHT FROM POUNDS TO KILOGRAMS

weight in pounds / 2.205 = weight in kg

Weight in lbs	Equation	Weight in kg
165	165 / 2.205	74.84 kg

CONVERT HEIGHT FROM FEET AND INCHES TO CENTIMETERS

(feet × 12 + inches) × 2.54 = height in cm

Height in feet and inches	Equation	Height in cm
5 ft 10 in	(5 × 12 + 10) × 2.54	177.8 cm

Next, we plug the values into:

MIFFLIN-ST. JEOR EQUATION FOR BMR FOR MEN

BMR (kcal/day) = (10 × weight in kg) + (6.25 × height in cm) − (5 × age in years) + 5

BMR = (10 × 74.84) + (6.25 × 177.8) − (5 × 45) + 5

BMR = 748.4 + 1111.25 − 225 + 5

BMR = 1639.65 kcal/day

Therefore, the estimated BMR for Doug would be approximately 1,640 kilocalories per day using the Mifflin-St. Jeor equation.

Thomas

Finally, for Thomas we follow the same steps.

CONVERT WEIGHT FROM POUNDS TO KILOGRAMS

weight in pounds / 2.205 = weight in kg

Weight in lbs	Equation	Weight in kg
285	285 / 2.205	129.27 kg

CONVERT HEIGHT FROM FEET AND INCHES TO CENTIMETERS

(feet × 12 + inches) × 2.54 = height in cm

Height in feet and inches	Equation	Height in cm
6 ft 4 in	(6 × 12 + 4) × 2.54	193.04 cm

Then, we plug the values into:

MIFFLIN-ST. JEOR EQUATION FOR BMR FOR MEN

BMR (kcal/day) = (10 × weight in kg) + (6.25 × height in cm) − (5 × age in years) + 5

BMR = (10 × 129.27) + (6.25 × 193.04) − (5 × 18) + 5

BMR = 1292.7 + 1206.5 − 90 + 5

BMR = 2414.20 kcal/day

Therefore, the estimated BMR for Thomas would be approximately 2,414 kilocalories per day using the Mifflin-St. Jeor equation.

Chapter 3

Jenny

Jenny would need 190 grams of carbohydrate in her pregame meal that is three-and-a-half hours away from activity. This is calculated by multiplying weight in kilograms by the number of hours until the activity (when between hours, round down).

63.50 kg × 3 = 190 g CHO

Doug

Doug would need 225 grams of carbohydrate in his pregame meal that is three hours away from activity.

74.84 kg × 3 = 225 g CHO

Thomas

Thomas would need 390 grams of carbohydrate in his pregame meal that is three-and-a-half hours away from activity.

129.27 kg × 3 = 390 g CHO

Chapter 4

Jenny

Jenny should aim for approximately 89 to 102 grams of protein per day. Because soccer involves both endurance and explosive movements, this was calculated by taking the middle ground of the two protein recommendation categories in table 4.2—a range of 1.4 to 1.6 grams per kilogram per day.

63.50 kg × 1.4 = 88.90 g PRO
63.50 kg × 1.6 = 101.60 g PRO

Doug

Doug should aim for 90 to 105 grams of protein per day. This is calculated by using the recommendation for endurance athletes of 1.2 to 1.4 grams per kilogram per day.

74.84 kg × 1.2 = 90 g PRO
74.84 kg × 1.4 = 105 g PRO

Thomas

Thomas should aim for 207 to 220 grams of protein per day. This is calculated by taking the recommendation for strength-based athletes of 1.6 to 1.7 grams per kilogram per day.

129.27 kg × 1.6 = 207 g PRO
129.27 kg × 1.7 = 220 g PRO

Chapter 7

Jenny

Jenny needs between 70 and 140 ounces of fluid per day. We calculate this by using the recommendation of 0.5 to 1 fluid ounce per pound of body weight.

140 lbs × 0.5 = 70 fl oz
140 lbs × 1 = 140 fl oz

Doug

Doug needs between 83 and 165 ounces of fluid per day.

165 lbs × 0.5 = 83 fl oz
165 lbs × 1 = 165 fl oz

Thomas

Thomas needs between 143 and 285 ounces of fluid per day.

285 lbs × 0.5 = 143 fl oz
285 lbs × 1 = 285 fl oz

Chapter 9

Jenny

If Jenny were having a pregame meal four hours before activity, she would want to aim for about 250 grams of carbohydrate. This is calculated by multiplying weight in kilograms by the number of hours until the activity.

63.50 kg × 4 = 254 g CHO

Doug

If Doug were having a prerace meal three hours before activity, he would want to aim for 225 grams of carbohydrate.

74.84 kg × 3 = 225 g CHO

Thomas

If Thomas were having a pregame meal three-and-a-half hours before activity, he should aim for around 390 grams of carbohydrate. Remember, when between hours, round down.

129.27 kg × 3 = 388 g CHO

Chapter 10

Doug

Doug would be classified as an endurance athlete, and depending on the volume of his training, he would fall into one of the following two ranges shown in table 10.1:

Moderate- to high-intensity endurance training, 1-3 hr/day 6-10 g/kg CHO

Moderate- to high-intensity endurance training, 4-5 hr/day 8-12 g/kg CHO

If he trained three hours per day, Doug would need on the higher end of the 6 to 10 grams per kilogram range. At 10 grams per kilogram, Doug would need 750 grams of carbohydrate per day.

74.84 kg × 10 = 750 g CHO/day

Chapter 11

Jenny

As a soccer player, Jenny would need between 6 and 10 grams per kilogram of carbohydrate per day; the exact amount would depend on her training and how many minutes she was playing during games. If she trained a couple of hours per day at a moderately high intensity, around 7 grams per kilogram of carbohydrate per day would be a good recommendation, so Jenny would need approximately 445 grams of carbohydrate per day.

$$63.50 \text{ kg} \times 7 = 445 \text{ g CHO/day}$$

Thomas

As a football player, Thomas would need between 5 and 7 grams per kilogram of carbohydrate per day; the exact amount would depend on his training and how many snaps he was getting in practice and on game days. Football games are very long (3-5 hours), so while the sport of football does not have a strong endurance component, the length of the activity can warrant higher carbohydrate intake, especially on game day. Around 6 grams per kilogram of carbohydrate for a game day would be a good recommendation, so Thomas would need 776 grams of carbohydrate on a game day. This amount might be lower on a training day.

$$129.27 \text{ kg} \times 6 = 776 \text{ g CHO/day}$$

References

CHAPTER 1

Arent, S.M., H.P. Cintineo, B.A. McFadden, A.J. Chandler, and M.A. Arent. 2020. "Nutrient Timing: A Garage Door of Opportunity?" *Nutrients* 12(7): 1948.

Biolo, G., K.D. Tipton, S. Klein, and R.R. Wolfe. 1997. "An Abundant Supply of Amino Acids Enhances the Metabolic Effect of Exercise on Muscle Protein." *American Journal of Physiology* 273, E122-E129.

Casa, D.J., L.E. Armstrong S.K. Hillman, et al. 2000. "National Athletic Trainers' Association Position Statement: Fluid Replacement for Athletes." *Journal of Athletic Training* 35 (2): 212–224.

Galloway, S.D., M.J. Lott, and L.C. Toulouse. 2014. "Preexercise Carbohydrate Feeding and High-Intensity Exercise Capacity: Effects of Timing of Intake and Carbohydrate Concentration." *International Journal of Sport Nutrition and Exercise Metabolism* 24 (3): 258–266.

Howarth, K.R., N.A. Moreau, S.M. Phillips, and M.J. Gibala. 2009. "Coingestion of Protein With Carbohydrate During Recovery From Endurance Exercise Stimulates Skeletal Muscle Protein Synthesis in Humans." *Journal of Applied Physiology (1985)* 106, no. 4 (April): 1394–1402.

Phillips, Stuart M., and Luc J.C. Van Loon. 2011. "Dietary Protein for Athletes: From Requirements to Optimum Adaptation." *Journal of Sports Sciences* 29, suppl. 1, S29-S38.

Tipton, K.D., D.L. Hamilton, and I.J. Gallagher. 2018. "Assessing the Role of Muscle Protein Breakdown in Response to Nutrition and Exercise in Humans." *Sports Medicine* 48, suppl. 1 (March): 53–64.

Vigh-Larsen, J.F., N. Ørtenblad, L.L. Spriet, K. Overgaard, and M. Mohr. 2021. "Muscle Glycogen Metabolism and High-Intensity Exercise Performance: A Narrative Review." *Sports Medicine* 51, 1855–1874.

Willoughby, D.S., J.R. Stout, and C.D. Wilborn. 2007. "Effects of Resistance Training and Protein Plus Amino Acid Supplementation on Muscle Anabolism, Mass, and Strength." *Amino Acids* 32 (4): 467–477.

CHAPTER 2

Link, L. 2018. *The Healthy Former Athlete: Nutrition and Fitness Advice for the Transition from Elite Athlete to Normal Human.* Skyhorse Publishing.

Mifflin, M.D., S.T. St. Jeor, L.A. Hill, B.J. Scott, S.A. Daugherty, and Y.O. Koh. 1990. "A New Predictive Equation for Resting Energy Expenditure in Healthy Individuals." *American Journal of Clinical Nutrition* 51 (2): 241–247.

Pontzer, H., Y. Yamada, H. Sagayama, P.N. Ainslie, L.F. Andersen, L.J. Anderson, L. Arab, I. Baddou, K. Bedu-Addo, E.E. Blaak, S. Blanc, A.G. Bonomi, C.V.C. Bouten, P. Bovet, M.S. Buchowski, N.F. Butte, S.G. Camps, G.L. Close, J.A. Cooper, R. Cooper, S.K. Das, L.R. Dugas, U. Ekelund, S. Entringer, T. Forrester, B.W. Fudge, A.H. Goris, M. Gurven, C. Hambly, A. El Hamdouchi, M.B. Hoos, S. Hu, N. Joonas, A.M. Joosen, P. Katzmarzyk, K.P. Kempen, M. Kimura, W.E. Kraus, R.F. Kushner, E.V. Lambert, W.R. Leonard, N. Lessan, C. Martin, A.C. Medin, E.P. Meijer, J.C. Morehen, J.P. Morton, M.L. Neuhouser, T.A. Nicklas, R.M. Ojiambo, K.H. Pietiläinen, Y.P.

Pitsiladis, J. Plange-Rhule, G. Plasqui, R.L. Prentice, R.A. Rabinovich, S.B. Racette, D.A. Raichlen, E. Ravussin, R.M. Reynolds, S.B. Roberts, A.J. Schuit, A.M. Sjödin, E. Stice, S.S. Urlacher, G. Valenti, L.M. Van Etten, E.A. Van Mil, J.C.K. Wells, G. Wilson, B.M. Wood, J. Yanovski, T. Yoshida, X. Zhang, A.J. Murphy-Alford, C. Loechl, A.H. Luke, J. Rood, D.A. Schoeller, K.R. Westerterp, W.W. Wong, J.R. Speakman. 2021. "Daily energy expenditure through the human life course." *Science* 373, no. 6556 (August 13): 808–812.

CHAPTER 3

Aragon, A.A., and B.J. Schoenfeld. 2013. "Nutrient Timing Revisited: Is There a Post-Exercise Anabolic Window?" *Journal of the International Society of Sports Nutrition* 10 (1): 1–13.

Burke, L.M., G.R. Cox, N.K. Culmmings, and B. Desbrow. 2001. "Guidelines for Daily Carbohydrate Intake: Do Athletes Achieve Them?" *Sports Medicine* 31 (4): 267–299.

Burke, L.M., J.A. Hawley, D.J. Angus, G.R. Cox, S.A. Clark, N.K. Cummings, B. Desbrow, et al. 2002. "Adaptations to Short-Term High-Fat Diet Persist During Exercise Despite High Carbohydrate Availability." *Medicine & Science in Sports & Exercise* 34 (1): 83–91.

Burke, L.M., J.A. Hawley, E.J. Schabort, A. St Clair Gibson, I. Mujika, and T.D. Noakes. 2000. "Carbohydrate Loading Failed to Improve 100-km Cycling Performance in a Placebo-Controlled Trial." *Journal of Applied Physiology (1985)* 88, no. 4 (April): 1284–1290.

Burke, L.M., M.L. Ross, L.A. Garvican-Lewis, M. Welvaert, I.A. Heikura, S.G. Forbes, J.G. Mirtschin, et al. 2017. "Low Carbohydrate, High Fat Diet Impairs Exercise Economy and Negates the Performance Benefit From Intensified Training in Elite Race Walkers." *Journal of Physiology* 595 (9): 2785–2807.

Coyle, E.F., A.R. Coggan, M.K. Hemmert, and J.L. Ivy. 1986. "Muscle Glycogen Utilization During Prolonged Strenuous Exercise When Fed Carbohydrate." *Journal of Applied Physiology* 61 (1): 165–172.

Haff, G.G., M.J. Lehmkuhl, L.B. McCoy, and M.H. Stone. 2003. "Carbohydrate Supplementation and Resistance Training." *Journal of Strength and Conditioning Research* 17, no. 1 (February): 187–196.

Ivy, J.L., A.L. Katz, C.L. Cutler, W.M. Sherman, and E.F. Coyle. 1985. "Muscle Glycogen Synthesis After Exercise: Effect of Time of Carbohydrate Ingestion." *Journal of Applied Physiology* 64, no. 4 (April): 1480–1485.

Jeukendrup, A. 2010. *Sports Nutrition: From Lab to Kitchen*. Aachen, Germany: Meyer & Meyer Sport.

Jentjens, R.L., and A.E. Jeukendrup. 2003. "Determinants of Post-Exercise Glycogen Synthesis During Short-Term Recovery." *Sports Medicine* 33 (2): 117–144.

Karpinski, C., and C.A. Rosenbloom, eds. 2017. *Sports Nutrition: A Handbook for Professionals*. 6th ed. New York: Academy of Nutrition and Dietetics.

Kerksick, C.M., S. Arent, B.J. Schoenfeld, J.R. Stout, B. Campbell, C.D. Wilborn, L. Taylor, et al. 2017. "International Society of Sports Nutrition Position Stand: Nutrient Timing." *Journal of the International Society of Sports Nutrition* 29, no. 14 (August): 33.

Nédélec, M., S. Halson, A.E. Abaidia, S. Ahmaidi, and G. Dupont. 2015. "Stress, Sleep and Recovery in Elite Soccer: A Critical Review of the Literature." *Sports Medicine* 45 (10): 1387–1400.

CHAPTER 4

Areta, J.L., L.M. Burke, M.L. Ross, D.M. Camera, D.W. West, E.M. Broad, N.A. Jeacocke, et al. 2013. "Timing and Distribution of Protein Ingestion During Prolonged Recovery From Resistance Exercise Alters Myofibrillar Protein Synthesis." *Journal of Physiology* 591, no. 9 (May 1): 2319–2331. doi: 10.1113/jphysiol.2012.244897. Epub 2013 Mar 4. PMID: 23459753; PMCID: PMC3650697.

Beelen, M., Zorenc, A., Pennings, B., Senden, J.M., Kuipers, H., van Loon, L.J. "Impact of protein coingestion on muscle protein synthesis during continuous endurance type exercise." *American Journal of Physiology-Endocrinology Metabolism.* 2011 Jun; 300(6):E945-54.

Biolo, G., K.D. Tipton, S. Klein, and R.R. Wolfe. 1997. "An Abundant Supply of Amino Acids Enhances the Metabolic Effect of Exercise on Muscle Protein." *American Journal of Physiology* 273, E122-E129.

Cribb, P.J., and A. Hayes. 2006. "Effects of Supplement Timing and Resistance Exercise on Skeletal Muscle Hypertrophy." *Medicine & Science in Sports & Exercise* 38, no. 11 (November): 1918–1925.

Hudson, J.L., R.E. Bergia, and W.W. Campbell. 2020. Protein distribution and muscle-related outcomes: Does the evidence support the concept? *Nutrients* 12, no. 5: 1441.

Jäger, R., Kerksick, C.M., Campbell, B.I., Cribb, P.J. "International Society of Sports Nutrition Position Stand: protein and exercise." *Journal of the International Society of Sports Nutrition.* 2017 Jun 20;14:20.

Karpinski, C., and C.A. Rosenbloom, eds. 2017. *Sports Nutrition: A Handbook for Professionals.* 6th ed. New York: Academy of Nutrition and Dietetics.

MacDougall, J.D., M.A. Tarnopolsky, A. Chesley, and S.A. Atkinson. 1992. "Changes in Muscle Protein Synthesis Following Heavy Resistance Exercise in Humans: A Pilot Study." *Acta Physiologica Scandinavica* 146, no. 3 (November): 403–404.

Mamerow, M.M., J.A. Mettler, K.L. English, S.L. Casperson, E. Arentson-Lantz, M. Sheffield-Moore, D.K. Layman, et al. 2014. "Dietary Protein Distribution Positively Influences 24-h Muscle Protein Synthesis in Healthy Adults." *The American Journal of Clinical Nutrition* 144 (6): 876–880.

Norton, L.E., and D.K. Layman. 2006. "Leucine Regulates Translation Initiation of Protein Synthesis in Skeletal Muscle After Exercise." *The Journal of Nutrition* 136 (2): 533S-537S.

Phillips, S.M., and L.J. Van Loon. 2011. "Dietary Protein for Athletes: From Requirements to Optimum Adaptation." *Journal of Sports Sciences* 29, suppl. 1, S29-S38.

Rennie, M.J., R.H. Edwards, D. Halliday, D.E. Matthews, S.L. Wolman, and D.J. Millward. 1982. "Muscle Protein Synthesis Measured by Stable Isotope Techniques in Man: The Effects of Feeding and Fasting." *Clinical Science* 63, no. 6 (December): 519–523.

Schoenfeld, B.J., A.A. Aragon, and J.W. Krieger. 2013. "The Effect of Protein Timing on Muscle Strength and Hypertrophy: A Meta-Analysis." *Journal of the International Society of Sports Nutrition* 10 (1): 53.

Tang, J.E., D.R. Moore, G.W. Kujbida, M.A. Tarnopolsky, and S.M. Phillips. 2009. "Ingestion of Whey Hydrolysate, Casein, or Soy Protein Isolate: Effects on Mixed Muscle Protein Synthesis at Rest and Following Resistance Exercise in Young Men." *Journal of Applied Physiology* 107 (3): 987–992.

Tipton, K.D., T.A. Elliott, M.G. Cree, A.A. Aarsland, A.P. Sanford, and R.R. Wolfe. 2007. "Stimulation of Net Muscle Protein Synthesis by Whey Protein Ingestion Before and

After Exercise." *American Journal of Physiology – Endocrinology and Metabolism* 292, no. 1 (January): E71-E76.

CHAPTER 5

American Heart Association. 2017. "Trans Fats." Accessed May 17, 2023, www.heart.org /en/healthy-living/healthy-eating/eat-smart/fats/trans-fat.

American Heart Association. 2021a. "Dietary Fats." Healthy Eating. Accessed May 17, 2023, www.heart.org/en/healthy-living/healthy-eating/eat-smart/fats/dietary-fats.

American Heart Association. 2021b. "Saturated Fats." Accessed May 17, 2023, www .heart.org/en/healthy-living/healthy-eating/eat-smart/fats/saturated-fats.

Calder, P.C. 2013. "N-3 Fatty Acids, Inflammation and Immunity: New Mechanisms to Explain Old Actions." *Proceedings of the Nutrition Society* 72, no. 3 (August): 326–336.

Impey, S.G., K.M. Hammond, S.O. Shepherd, A.P. Sharples, C. Stewart, M. Limb, K. Smith, et al. 2016. "Fuel for the Work Required: A Practical Approach to Amalgamating Train-Low Paradigms for Endurance Athletes." *Physiological Reports* 4 (10): e12803.

Institute of Medicine. 2002. *Dietary Reference Intakes for Energy, Carbohydrate, Fiber, Fat, Fatty Acids, Cholesterol, Protein, and Amino Acids.* Washington, DC: National Academies Press.

Mensink, R.P., P.L. Zock, A.D. Kester, and M.B. Katan. 2003. "Effects of Dietary Fatty Acids and Carbohydrates on the Ratio of Serum Total to HDL Cholesterol and on Serum Lipids and Apolipoproteins: A Meta-Analysis of 60 Controlled Trials." *American Journal of Clinical Nutrition* 77, no. 5 (May): 1146–1155.

National Institutes of Health. 2023. "Omega-3 Fatty Acids: Fact Sheet for Health Professionals." https://ods.od.nih.gov/factsheets/Omega3FattyAcids-HealthProfessional.

Paoli, A., A. Bianco, K.A. Grimaldi, A. Lodi, and G. Bosco. 2013. "Long Term Successful Weight Loss With a Combination Biphasic Ketogenic Mediterranean Diet and Mediterranean Diet Maintenance Protocol." *Nutrients* 5 (12): 5205–5217.

Rowlands, D.S., and W.G. Hopkins. 2002. "Effects of High-Fat and High-Carbohydrate Diets on Metabolism and Performance in Cycling." *Metabolism* 51, no. 6 (June): 678–690.

Simopoulos, A.P. 2002. *"The Importance of the Ratio of Omega-6/Omega-3 Essential Fatty Acids."* Biomed Pharmacotherapy 56, no. 8 (October): 365–79.

Tomten, S.E., and A.T. Høstmark. 2006. "Energy Balance in Weight Stable Athletes With and Without Menstrual Disorders." *Scandinavian Journal of Medicine and Science in Sports* 16, no. 2 (April): 127–133.

Volek, J.S., D.J. Freidenreich, C. Saenz, L.J. Kunces, B.C. Creighton, J.M. Bartley, P.M. Davitt, et al. 2016. "Metabolic Characteristics of Keto-Adapted Ultra-Endurance Runners." *Metabolism* 65, no. 3: 100–110.

Whittaker, J., K. Wu. 2021. "Low-Fat Diets and Testosterone in Men: Systematic Review and Meta-Analysis of Intervention Studies." *Journal of Steroid Biochemistry and Molecular Biology* 210, no. 105878 (June).

Wynne, J.L., A.M. Ehlert, P.B. Wilson. 2021. "Effects of High-Carbohydrate Versus Mixed-Macronutrient Meals on Female Soccer Physiology and Performance." *European Journal of Applied Physiology* 4, no. 121 (April): 1125–1134.

Yeo, W.K., A.L. Carey, L. Burke, L.L. Spriet, and J.A. Hawley. 2011. "Fat Adaptation in Well-Trained Athletes: Effects on Cell Metabolism." *Applied Physiology, Nutrition, and Metabolism* 36, no. 1 (February): 12–22.

Zajac, A., S. Poprzecki, A. Maszczyk, M. Czuba, M. Michalczyk, and G. Zydek. 2014. "The Effects of a Ketogenic Diet on Exercise Metabolism and Physical Performance in Off-Road Cyclists." *Nutrients* 6 (7): 2493–2508.

CHAPTER 6

Arab, A., N. Rafie, R. Amani, and F. Shirani. 2022. "The Role of Magnesium in Sleep Health: A Systematic Review of Available Literature." *Biological Trace Element Research* 201 (1): 121–128.

Benardot, D. 2021. *Advanced Sports Nutrition*. 3rd ed. Champaign, IL: Human Kinetics.

Braakhuis, A.J., W.G. Hopkins, and T.E. Lowe. 2013. "Effect of Dietary Antioxidants, Training, and Performance Correlates on Antioxidant Status in Competitive Rowers." *International Journal of Sports Physiology and Performance* 8, no. 5 (September): 565–572.

Braam, L.A., M.H. Knapen, P. Geusens, F. Brouns, K. Hamulyák, M.J. Gerichhausen, and C. Vermeer. 2003. "Vitamin K1 Supplementation Retards Bone Loss in Post-menopausal Women Between 50 and 60 Years of Age." *Calcified Tissue International* 73, no. 1 (July): 21–26. doi: 10.1007/s00223-002-2084-4. PMID: 14506950.

Harvard School of Public Health. n.d. "Salt and Sodium." www.hsph.harvard.edu/nutritionsource/salt-and-sodium. Accessed February 23, 2023.

Institute of Medicine. 2001. *Dietary Reference Intakes for Vitamin A, Vitamin K, Arsenic, Boron, Chromium, Copper, Iodine, Iron, Manganese, Molybdenum, Nickel, Silicon, Vanadium, and Zinc*. Washington DC: National Academies Press. www.ncbi.nlm.nih.gov/books/NBK222310.

Jiang, Q. 2014. "Natural Forms of Vitamin E: Metabolism, Antioxidant, and Anti-Inflammatory Activities and Their Role in Disease Prevention and Therapy." *Free Radical Biology and Medicine* 72, 76–90.

Kilic, M., A.K. Baltaci, M. Gunay, H. Gökbel, N. Okudan, and I. Cicioglu. 2006. "The Effect of Exhaustion Exercise on Thyroid Hormones and Testosterone Levels of Elite Athletes Receiving Oral Zinc." *Neuroendocrinology Letters* 27, no. 1–2 (February-April): 247–252.

Manore, M.M. 2000. "Effect of Physical Activity on Thiamine, Riboflavin, and Vitamin B-6 Requirements." *American Journal of Clinical Nutrition* 72, suppl. 2, 598S-606S.

National Institutes of Health. n.d. "Nutrient Recommendations: Dietary Reference Intakes (DRI)." https://ods.od.nih.gov/HealthInformation/nutrientrecommendations.aspx.

Paulsen, G., K.T. Cumming, G. Holden, J. Hallén, B.R. Rønnestad, O. Sveen, A. Skaug, i. Paur, N.E. Bastani, H.N. Østgaard, C. Buer, M. Midttun, F. Freuchen, H. Wiig, E.T. Ulseth, I. Garthe, R. Blomhoff, H.B. Benestad, T. Raastad. 2014. "Vitamin C and E Supplementation Hampers Cellular Adaptation to Endurance Training in Humans: A Double-blind, Randomised, Controlled Trial." *Journal of Physiology*, 592 (8): 1887-901.

Reno, A.M., M. Green, L.G. Killen, E.K. O'Neal, K. Pritchett, and Z. Hanson. 2022. "Effects of Magnesium Supplementation on Muscle Soreness and Performance." *Journal of Strength and Conditioning Research* 36 (8): 2198–2203.

Renzi-Hammond, L.M., E.R. Bovier, L.M. Fletcher, L.S. Miller, C.M. Mewborn, C.A. Lindbergh, J.H. Baxter, et al. 2017. "Effects of a Lutein and Zeaxanthin Intervention on Cognitive Function: A Randomized, Double-Masked, Placebo-Controlled Trial of Younger Healthy Adults." *Nutrients* 9, no. 11 (November 14): 1246.

Sanders, K.M., G.C. Nicholson, and P.R. Ebeling. 2012. "Is High Dose Vitamin D Harmful?" *Calcified Tissue International* 92 (2): 191–206.

Sato, A., Y. Shimoyama, T. Ishikawa, and N. Murayama. 2011. "Dietary Thiamin and Riboflavin Intake and Blood Thiamin and Riboflavin Concentrations in College Swimmers Undergoing Intensive Training." *International Journal of Sport Nutrition and Exercise Metabolism* 21 (3): 195–204.

Wessels, I., M. Maywald, and L. Rink. 2017. "Zinc as a Gatekeeper of Immune Function." *Nutrients* 9, no. 12 (November 25): 1286.

CHAPTER 7

Adan, A. 2012. "Cognitive Performance and Dehydration." *Journal of the American College of Nutrition* 31, no. 2 (April): 71–78.

Garvican-Lewis, L.A., A.D. Govus, P. Peeling, C.R. Abbiss, and C.J. Gore. 2016. "Iron Supplementation and Altitude: Decision Making Using a Regression Tree." *Journal of Sports Science and Medicine* 15 (1), 204–205.

Goulet, E.D. 2012. "Dehydration and Endurance Performance in Competitive Athletes." *Nutrition Reviews* 70, suppl. 2 (November): S132-S136.

Hew-Butler, T., M.H. Rosner, S. Fowkes-Godek, J.P. Dugas, M.D. Hoffman, D.P. Lewis, and R.J. Maughan, et al. 2015. "Statement of the Third International Exercise-Associated Hyponatremia Consensus Development Conference, Carlsbad, California." *Clinical Journal of Sport Medicine* 25, no. 4 (July): 303–320.

Knechtle, B., T. Rosemann, and P.T. Nikolaidis. 2018. "Pacing and Changes in Body Composition in 48 h Ultra-Endurance Running: A Case Study." *Sports (Basel)* 6, no. 4 (November 1): 136. doi: 10.3390/sports6040136. PMID: 30388759; PMCID: PMC6315888.

Miller, K.C., B.P. McDermott, S.W. Yeargin, A. Fiol, and M.P. Schwellnus. 2022. "An Evidence-Based Review of the Pathophysiology, Treatment, and Prevention of Exercise-Associated Muscle Cramps." *Journal of Athletic Training* 57, no. 1 (January 1): 5–15.

Saunders, P.U., L.A. Garvican-Lewis, R.F. Chapman, and J.D. Périard. 2019. "Special Environments: Altitude and Heat." *International Journal of Sport Nutrition and Exercise Metabolism* 29, no. 2 (March): 210–219.

Sawka, M.N. 1992. "Physiological Consequences of Hypohydration: Exercise Performance and Thermoregulation." *Medicine & Science in Sports & Exercise* 24, no. 6 (June): 657–670.

Sawka, M.N., L.M. Burke, E.R. Eichner, R.J. Maughan, S.J. Montain, and N.S. Stachenfeld. 2007. "American College of Sports Medicine Position Stand. Exercise and Fluid Replacement." *Medicine & Science in Sports & Exercise* 39, no. 2 (February): 377–390.

Schwellnus, M.P. 2009. "Cause of Exercise Associated Muscle Cramps (EAMC)—Altered Neuromuscular Control, Dehydration, or Electrolyte Depletion?" *British Journal of Sports Medicine* 43 (6): 401–408.

CHAPTER 8

Antonio, J., D.G. Candow, S.C. Forbes, B. Gualano, A.R. Jagim, R.B. Kreider, E.S. Rawson, et al. 2021. "Common Questions and Misconceptions About Creatine Supplementation: What Does the Scientific Evidence Really Show?" *Journal of the International Society of Sports Nutrition* 18, no. 1 (February 8): 13.

Bonilla, D.A., Y. Moreno, C. Gho, J.L. Petro, A. Odriozola-Martínez, R.B. Kreider. 2021. "Effects of Ashwagandha (*Withania somnifera*) on Physical Performance: Systematic Review and Bayesian Meta-Analysis." *Journal of Functional Morphology and Kinesiology* 6 (1): 20.

Candow, D.G., S.C. Forbes, M.D. Roberts, B.D. Roy, J. Antonio, A.E. Smith-Ryan, E.S. Rawson, et al. 2022. "Creatine O'Clock: Does Timing of Ingestion Really Influence Muscle Mass and Performance?" *Frontiers in Sports and Active Living* 4 (May 20): 893714.

Clark, K.L., W. Sebastianelli, K.R. Flechsenhar, D.F. Aukermann, F. Meza, R.L. Millard, and A. Albert. 2008. "24-Week Study on the Use of Collagen Hydrolysate as a Dietary Supplement in Athletes With Activity-Related Joint Pain." *Current Medical Research and Opinion* 24(5): 1485–1496.

Crawford, C., B. Avula, A.T. Lindsey, A. Walter, K. Katragunta, I.A. Khan, and P.A. Deuster. 2022. "Analysis of Select Dietary Supplement Products Marketed to Support or Boost the Immune System." *JAMA Network Open* 5, no. 8 (Aug 1): e2226040.

De Bock, K., B.O. Eijnde, M. Ramaekers, and P. Hespel. 2004. "Acute Rhodiola Rosea Intake Can Improve Endurance Exercise Performance." *International Journal of Sport Nutrition and Exercise Metabolism* 14: 298–307.

Dolan, E., B. Gualano, E.S. Rawson. 2019. "Beyond Muscle: The Effects of Creatine Supplementation on Brain Creatine, Cognitive Processing, and Traumatic Brain Injury." *European Journal of Sport Science* 19 (1): 1–14.

Forbes, S.C., D.M. Cordingley, S.M. Cornish, B. Gualano, H. Roschel, S.M. Ostojic, E.S. Rawson, et al. 2022. "Effects of Creatine Supplementation on Brain Function and Health." *Nutrients* 14, no. 5 (February 22): 921.

Gonzalez, A.M., and E.T. Trexler. 2020. "Effects of Citrulline Supplementation on Exercise Performance in Humans: A Review of the Current Literature." *Journal of Strength and Conditioning Research* May;34(5):1480–1495.

Grgic, J., F. Sabol, S. Venier, I. Mikulic, N. Bratkovic, B.J. Schoenfeld, C. Pickering, et al. 2019. "What Dose of Caffeine to Use: Acute Effects of 3 Doses of Caffeine on Muscle Endurance and Strength." *International Journal of Sports Physiology and Performance* (September 9): 1–8.

Guest, N.S., T.A. VanDusseldorp, M.T. Nelson, J. Grgic, B.J. Schoenfeld, N.D.M. Jenkins, S.M. Arent, et al. 2021. "International Society of Sports Nutrition Position Stand: Caffeine and Exercise Performance." *Journal of the International Society of Sports Nutrition* 18, 1. https://doi.org/10.1186/s12970-020-00383-4.

Jäger, R., M. Purpura, and M. Kingsley. 2007. "Phospholipids and Sports Performance." *Journal of the International Society of Sports Nutrition* 4, no. 5 (July 25). doi: 10.1186/1550-2783-4-5.

Kreider, R.B., D.S. Kalman, J. Antonio, T.N. Ziegenfuss, R. Wildman, R. Collins, D.G. Candow, et al. 2017. "International Society of Sports Nutrition Position Stand: Safety and Efficacy of Creatine Supplementation in Exercise, Sport, and Medicine." *Journal of the International Society of Sports Nutrition* 14 (June 13): 18.

Lane, S., J.A. Hawley, B. Desbrow, A.M. Jones, J.R. Blackwell, M.L. Ross, A.J. Zemski, et al. 2014. "Single and Combined Effects of Beetroot Juice and Caffeine Supplementation on Cycling Time Trial Performance." *Applied Physiology, Nutrition, and Metabolism* 39: 1050–1057.

Lewis, M.D. 2016. "Concussions, Traumatic Brain Injury, and the Innovative Use of Omega-3s." *Journal of the American College of Nutrition* 35, no. 5 (July): 469–475. doi: 10.1080/07315724.2016.1150796. PMID: 27454858.

Lugo, J.P., Z.M. Saiyed, F.C. Lau, J.P.L. Molina, M.N. Pakdaman, A.N. Shamie, and J.K. Udani. 2013. "Undenatured Type II Collagen (UC-II (R)) for Joint Support: A Randomized, Double-Blind, Placebo-Controlled Study in Healthy Volunteers." *Journal of the International Society of Sports Nutrition* 10 (1): 10–48.

Machek, S.B., and J.R. Bagley. 2018. "Creatine Monohydrate Supplementation: Considerations for Cognitive Performance in Athletes." *Strength & Conditioning Journal* 40 (2): 82–93.

McMahon, N.F., M.D. Leveritt, and T.G. Pavey. 2017. "The Effect of Dietary Nitrate Supplementation on Endurance Exercise Performance in Healthy Adults: A Systematic Review and Meta-Analysis." *Sports Medicine* 47 (4): 735–756.

Nelson, A.G., D.A. Arnall, J. Kokkonen, R. Day, J. Evans. 2001. "Muscle Glycogen Supercompensation Is Enhanced by Prior Creatine Supplementation." *Medicine and Science in Sports and Exercise* 33 33 (7): 1096–100.

Pérez-Gómez, J., S. Villafaina, J.C. Adsuar, E. Merellano-Navarro, and D. Collado-Mateo. 2020. "Effects of Ashwagandha (*Withania somnifera*) on VO_{2max}: A Systematic Review and Meta-Analysis." *Nutrients* 12 (4): 1119.

Philpott, J.D., C. Donnelly, I.H. Walshe, E.E. MacKinley, J. Dick, S.D.R. Galloway, K.D. Tipton, et al. 2018. "Adding Fish Oil to Whey Protein, Leucine, and Carbohydrate Over a Six-Week Supplementation Period Attenuates Muscle Soreness Following Eccentric Exercise in Competitive Soccer Players." *International Journal of Sport Nutrition and Exercise Metabolism* 28 (1): 26–36.

Philpott, J.D., O.C. Witard, and S.D.R. Galloway. 2019. "Applications of Omega-3 Polyunsaturated Fatty Acid Supplementation for Sport Performance." *Research in Sports Medicine* 27 (2): 219–237.

Saunders, B., K. Elliott-Sale, G.G. Artioli, P.A. Swinton, E. Dolan, H. Roschel, C. Sale, et al. 2017. "B-Alanine Supplementation to Improve Exercise Capacity and Performance: A Systematic Review and Meta-Analysis." *British Journal of Sports Medicine* 51, no. 8 (April): 658–669.

Schifano, F., V. Catalani, S. Sharif, F. Napoletano, J.M. Corkery, D. Arillotta, S. Fergus, et al. 2022. "Benefits and Harms of 'Smart Drugs' (Nootropics) in Healthy Individuals." *Drugs* 82, no. 6 (April): 633–647.

Senefeld, J.W., C.C. Wiggins, R.J. Regimbal, P.B. Dominelli, S.E. Baker, and M.J. Joyner. 2020. "Ergogenic Effect of Nitrate Supplementation: A Systematic Review and Meta-Analysis." *Medicine & Science in Sports & Exercise* 52, no.10 (October): 2250–2261.

Shaw, G., A. Lee-Barthel, M.L. Ross, B. Wang, and K. Baar. 2017. "Vitamin C-Enriched Gelatin Supplementation Before Intermittent Activity Augments Collagen Synthesis." *American Journal of Clinical Nutrition* 105, no. 1 (January): 136–143. doi: 10.3945/ajcn.116.138594. Epub 2016 Nov 16. PMID: 27852613; PMCID: PMC5183725.

Stecker, R.A., P.S. Harty, A.R. Jagim, D.G. Candow, and C.M. Kerksick. 2019. "Timing of Ergogenic Aids and Micronutrients on Muscle and Exercise Performance." *Journal of the International Society of Sports Nutrition* 16, no. 1 (September 2): 37.

Tan, R., L. Cano, Á. Lago-Rodríguez, and R. Domínguez. 2022. "The Effects of Dietary Nitrate Supplementation on Explosive Exercise Performance: A Systematic Review." *International Journal of Environmental Research and Public Health* 19, no. 2 (January 11): 762.

Therapeutic Research Center. 2023. "Natural Medicines Database: Caffeine." https://naturalmedicines.therapeuticresearch.com/databases/food,-herbs-supplements/professional.aspx?productid=979#safety. Accessed May 2022, 2023. Therapeutic Research Center. 2023. "Natural Medicines Database: Panax Ginseng." https://naturalmedicines.therapeuticresearch.com/databases/food,-herbs-supplements/professional.aspx?productid=1000#scientificName. Accessed May 15, 2023.

Therapeutic Research Center. 2023. "Natural Medicines Database: Gingko." https://naturalmedicines.therapeuticresearch.com/databases/food,-herbs-supplements/professional.aspx?productid=333#scientificName. Accessed May 15, 2023.

Therapeutic Research Center. 2023. "Natural Medicines Database: Rhodiola." https://naturalmedicines.therapeuticresearch.com/databases/food,-herbs-supplements/professional.aspx?productid=883#scientificName. Accessed June 1, 2023.

Therapeutic Research Center. 2023. "Natural Medicines Database: Phosphatidylcholine." https://naturalmedicines.therapeuticresearch.com/databases/food,-herbs-supplements/professional.aspx?productid=501. Accessed July 11, 2023.

Van Cutsem, J., K. De Pauw, S. Marcora, R. Meeusen, and B. Roelands. 2018. "A Caffeine-Maltodextrin Mouth Rinse Counters Mental Fatigue." *Psychopharmacology (Berl)* 235, no. 4 (April): 947–958.

CHAPTER 10

Burke, L.M. 2021. "Ketogenic Low-CHO, High-Fat Diet: The Future of Elite Endurance Sport?" *Journal of Physiology* 599, no. 3 (February): 819–843.

Burke, L.M., J. Whitfield, I.A. Heikura, M.L.R. Ross, N. Tee, S.F. Forbes, R. Hall, et al. 2021. "Adaptation to a Low Carbohydrate High Fat Diet Is Rapid but Impairs Endurance Exercise Metabolism and Performance Despite Enhanced Glycogen Availability." *Journal of Physiology* 599, no. 3 (February): 771–790.

Chapman-Lopez, T.J., and Y. Koh. 2022. "The Effects of Medium-Chain Triglyceride Oil Supplementation on Endurance Performance and Substrate Utilization in Healthy Populations: A Systematic Review." *Journal of Obesity and Metabolic Syndrome* 31, no. 3 (September 30): 217–229.

Fairchild, T.J., S. Fletcher, P. Steele, C. Goodman, B. Dawson, and P.A. Fournier. 2002. "Rapid Carbohydrate Loading After a Short Bout of Near Maximal-Intensity Exercise." *Medicine & Science in Sports & Exercise* 34, no. 6 (June): 980–986.

Kato, H., K. Suzuki, M. Bannai, and D.R. Moore. 2016. "Protein Requirements Are Elevated in Endurance Athletes Sfter Exercise as Determined by the Indicator Amino Acid Oxidation Method." *PLoS One* 11, no. 6 (June 20): e0157406.

Wismann, J., and D. Willoughby. 2006. "Gender Differences in Carbohydrate Metabolism and Carbohydrate Loading." *Journal of the International Society of Sports Nutrition* 3, no. 1 (June): 28–34.

CHAPTER 12

Ainsley Dean, P.J., G. Arikan, B. Opitz, and A. Sterr. 2017. "Potential for Use of Creatine Supplementation Following Mild Traumatic Brain Injury." *Concussion* 2 (2): CNC34.

Barchitta, M., A. Maugeri, G. Favara, R. Magnano San Lio, G. Evola, A. Agodi, and G. Basile. 2019. "Nutrition and Wound Healing: An Overview Focusing on the Beneficial Effects of Curcumin." *International Journal of Molecular Sciences* 20, no. 5 (March 5): 1119.

Barrett, E.C., M.I. McBurney, and E.D. Ciappio. 2014. "ω-3 Fatty Acid Supplementation as a Potential Therapeutic Aid for the Recovery from Mild Traumatic Brain Injury/Concussion." *Advances in Nutrition* 5 (3): 268–277.

Hirsch, K.R., R.R. Wolfe, and A.A. Ferrando. 2021. "Pre- and Post-Surgical Nutrition for Preservation of Muscle Mass, Strength, and Functionality Following Orthopedic Surgery." *Nutrients* 13, no. 5 (May 15): 1675.

Lis, D.M., and K. Baar. 2019. "Effects of Different Vitamin C-Enriched Collagen Derivatives on Collagen Synthesis." *International Journal of Sport Nutrition and Exercise Metabolism* 29, no. 5 (September 1): 526–531.

Mishra, S., V.J. Singh, P.A. Chawla, and V. Chawla. 2022. "Neuroprotective Role of Nutritional Supplementation in Athletes." *Current Molecular Pharmacology* 15 (1): 129–142.

Oliver, J.M., A.J. Anzalone, and S.M. Turner. 2018. "Protection Before Impact: The Potential Neuroprotective Role of Nutritional Supplementation in Sports-Related Head Trauma." *Sports Medicine* 48, suppl. 1 (March): 39–52.

Shaw, G., A. Lee-Barthel, M.L. Ross, B. Wang, and K. Baar. 2017. "Vitamin C-Enriched Gelatin Supplementation Before Intermittent Activity Augments Collagen Synthesis." *American Journal of Clinical Nutrition* 105, no. 1 (January): 136–143.

Smith-Ryan, A.E., K.R. Hirsch, H.E. Saylor, L.M. Gould, and M.N.M. Blue. 2020. "Nutritional Considerations and Strategies to Facilitate Injury Recovery and Rehabilitation." *Journal of Athletic Training* 55, no. 9 (September 1): 918–930.

Tipton, K.D. 2015. "Nutritional Support for Exercise-Induced Injuries." *Sports Medicine* 45, suppl. 1 (November): S93–104.

Wu, A., Z. Ying, and F. Gomez-Pinilla. 2006. "Dietary Curcumin Counteracts the Outcome of Traumatic Brain Injury on Oxidative Stress, Synaptic Plasticity, and Cognition." *Experimental Neurology* 197 (2): 309–317.

Zhu, H.T., C. Bian, J.C. Yuan, W. Chu, X. Xiang, F. Chen, C. Wang, et al. 2014. "Curcumin Attenuates Acute Inflammatory Injury by Inhibiting the TLR4/MyD88/NF-κ\B Signaling Pathway in Experimental Traumatic Brain Injury." *Journal of Neuroinflammation* 11 (March): 59.

Index

About the Author

Lauren Link, MS, RD, CSSD, is an assistant athletics director and the director of sport nutrition for Purdue University Athletics, where she oversees the sport nutrition program and works with football, men's basketball, volleyball, and women's soccer. Her primary duties include providing individual and team nutrition education; providing counseling and medical nutrition therapy as needed; evaluating supplements for legality, safety, and efficacy; assessing body composition and identifying athletes at high risk for bone injury using Lunar iDXA technology; overseeing the fueling stations and athletic dining hall; and managing a seven-figure budget to provide all teams with appropriate nutrition.

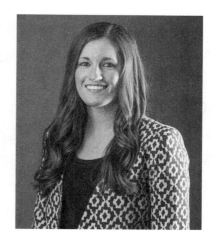

In addition to fueling her athletes for success on the playing field, she is also passionate about helping athletes successfully navigate the transition into the real world. She has led multiple initiatives to this end, founding the Purdue student-athlete community garden and spearheading a program called BLAST—for Boiler Life After Sport—designed to help address key components of athletes' transition to "normal" life. In 2017 she published her first book on the subject: *The Healthy Former Athlete*.

Link graduated from Purdue University with a bachelor of science degree in dietetics and health, nutrition, and fitness (December 2011) and a master of science degree in health and kinesiology (December 2019). She was a member of the Purdue women's soccer team from 2007 through 2011 and was part of the 2007 Big Ten tournament championship team. She is a registered dietitian (RD) and holds the Board-Certified Specialist in Sports Dietetics (CSSD) credential. She is active within the Collegiate and Professional Sports Dietitians Association (CPSDA) and is a member of the Sports and Human Performance Nutrition (SHPN) practice group.

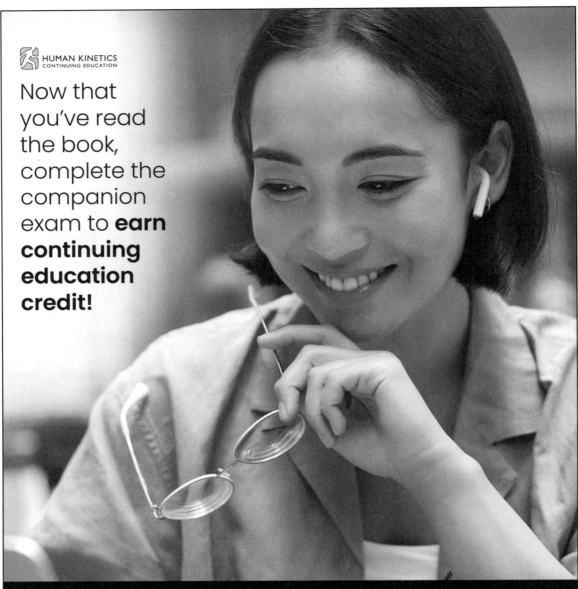
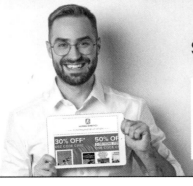